Strong Women, Strong Hearts

MIRIAM E. NELSON, PhD AND

ALICE H. LICHTENSTEIN, DSc

with

LAWRENCE LINDNER, MA

*Friedman School of Nutrition Science
and Policy, Tufts University, Boston, MA*

Strong Women, Strong Hearts

PROVEN STRATEGIES TO
PREVENT AND REDUCE
HEART DISEASE
NOW

Aurum

First published in Great Britain 2005
by Aurum Press Ltd
25 Bedford Avenue, London WC1B 3AT
Published by arrangement with Penguin Group (USA) Inc.

A catalogue record for this book is available from the British Library
ISBN 1 84513 105 3

1   3   5   7   9   10   8   6   4   2
2005   2007   2009   2008   2006

Printed by MPG Books, Bodmin, Cornwall

PAR-Q questionnaire on pages 104–105 reprinted with permission of Canada Society for Exercise Physiology.
    Exercise intensity scales on pages 114 and 118 used with permission from Miriam E. Nelson, PhD, with Sarah Wernick, PhD, *Strong Women Stay Young* (London: Aurum Press 2000).
    Select recipes on pages 94–96 used with permission from Miriam E. Nelson, PhD, with Judy Knipe, *Strong Women Eat Well* (G. P. Putnam's Sons, 2001).
    Illustrations by Wendy Wray/Vicki Morgan Associates, NYC.

    Neither the publisher nor the authors are engaged in rendering professional advice or services to the individual reader. The ideas, procedures and suggestions contained in this book are not intended as a substitute for consulting with your physician. All matters regarding your health require medical supervision. Neither the authors nor the publisher shall be liable or responsible for any loss or damage allegedly arising from any information or suggestion in this book.

    The recipes contained in this book are to be followed exactly as written. The publisher is not responsible for your specific health or allergy needs that may require medical supervision. The publisher is not responsible for any adverse reactions to the recipes contained in this book.

    Research is conducted at Tufts University with the expectation of publication. In such publication the authors alone are responsible for statements of fact, opinions, recommendations and conclusions expressed. Publication does not imply approval or endorsement by Tufts University.

An Important Caution

The advice given in *Strong Women, Strong Hearts* is based on extensive scientific research. This book contains instructions and safety precautions. It is essential that you read them carefully. Some exercises are inappropriate for individuals with heart disease or other medical conditions.

This book is not intended to replace the services of a general practitioner who knows you personally. An essential element of taking responsibility for your health is having regular checkups and working in partnership with medical professionals.

If you are under treatment for heart disease or any other medical condition – or if you suspect you might need such care – you must discuss this programme with your doctor before you begin.

Contents

---◆---

PART 3 ◆ Beyond Lifestyle

Preface

◆

Going on two years ago, I was walking into our research centre at Tufts University one day when a colleague, Dr Alice Lichtenstein, stopped me in the hallway. I had written books about osteoporosis, arthritis, weight control and other conditions, she said, but why hadn't I yet written *Strong Women, Strong Hearts*? After all, she argued, there is perhaps no more important impact that exercise and good nutrition have on health than to reduce the risk of heart disease. On top of that, Alice said, more women die of heart disease each year than men, but most women aren't aware of that. They need to hear about it and they need to learn what to do to avoid it.

She was right, of course. But I looked at her and responded, 'Alice, that's *your* book to write'. Alice is one of the world's finest scientists in the field of nutrition and heart disease; she heads the Cardiovascular Nutrition Laboratory at Tufts and currently chairs the Nutrition Committee of the American Heart Association.

'We need to talk,' she said. 'Without you and your expertise in physical activity, we don't have the crucial exercise component.'

A week later, I met with Alice to discuss collaborating on this book. And soon after that, we were putting together *Strong Women, Strong Hearts* with our collaborator, Larry Lindner, who brought his writing talent to bear on the project.

Preparing this book with Alice has been an incredibly rich experience, one that you might say was twenty years in the making. I remember very well when, as a graduate student in 1984, I listened enthralled on those days she appeared as a new-graduate guest lecturer in my nutritional biochemistry class. I remember being in awe of her command of the science, her ability to explain the intricacies of dietary fats and carbohydrates. I was fascinated by her explanations of what happens to food once it is absorbed; how it gets metabolized and increases or decreases the risk for chronic disease.

I am learning from Alice still. There was much I learned, in fact, during the writing of this book (and, she insisted I include here, much she learned from me).

We both hope that you learn, too, as you read – and are inspired to take steps to protect yourself. Premature death and disability from heart disease can be largely eliminated if women make the choice to eat better and exercise more.

From both Alice and me, here's to strong women – with very strong hearts.

Miriam Nelson

PART 1

Women and Heart Disease – Where Are We Now?

CHAPTER 1

A Call to Action

◆

I was first diagnosed with borderline high blood pressure in my twenties, when I was pregnant. I still had high blood pressure after I gave birth, but I was told only that I had to go on a strict diet even though I wasn't really overweight. I went like that for years, with my blood pressure getting higher and higher throughout my thirties. Not until I was in my forties and my blood pressure skyrocketed to 200 over 100 was I given medication to lower it.

— LINDA

I woke up one morning with severe chest pain, severe upper back pain, nauseated, short of breath – an overall horrible feeling. It got worse and worse throughout the day. Finally, I went to casualty. The doctor said, 'It's probably just a muscle . . . I'm going to give you a muscle relaxant and send you home.' But as much as I was rationalizing ('Did I play racquetball too hard? Could this be food poisoning?'), I had this sense of doom. I didn't want to leave until I had had further testing. 'I want an ECG,' I said. 'I want a blood test.' Reluctantly, they agreed. When they first attached me to the ECG machine, the nurse thought she had hooked me up wrong. She called in another nurse. Then they got the doctor. It took twenty minutes for them to finally believe I was having a heart attack.

— CINDY

I had to wait thirty minutes in casualty. They thought I had indigestion and sent me home with very strong pain medication. I was back in the emergency department late that night. They finally did an ECG – and immediately air-lifted me to a larger hospital for emergency heart surgery. I stopped breathing on the operating table.

– DeLinda

HEART DISEASE KILLS MORE WOMEN THAN MEN

Unfortunately, what happened to these women is not unique. Heart disease is considered a man's problem, but every year since 1984, it has killed more women than men in the United States. A woman dies from heart disease about once every minute, for an annual total of about half a million deaths. There are also lots of women *living* with heart disease – some eight million in the US.

It has clearly reached a crisis point, one that reflects an unfortunate irony. So much has been made of women's hearts as symbols – of love, purity of emotion, the centre of a home. But the female heart can become diseased and the very realness of the heart as giver of life is ignored.

Even if a woman *is* properly diagnosed, she is often not properly tended to:

- Whereas 25 per cent of men die within one year of a first heart attack, the number surges to 38 per cent for women.
- Eighteen per cent of male heart attack survivors experience a second heart attack within six years, compared with 35 per cent of women heart attack sufferers – almost twice the proportion.
- Women are almost two times as likely as men to die after bypass surgery and half as likely to get an angioplasty to open a narrowed blood vessel.

Unfortunately, stubborn myths about women and heart disease stand in the way of effective treatment.

Myth: When it comes to women, it's more important to focus on breast cancer than heart disease.

Fact: Heart disease is the leading killer of women in the United States, taking many times more lives than breast cancer. Breast cancer is a devastating disease, but you can't deny the numbers. Heart disease kills 499,000 women each year (compared with 432,000 men). Breast cancer kills 40,000 women each year.

Myth: It's men who need to be the focus of lifestyle changes for preventing heart disease.

Fact: Women need to protect themselves by living heart-heathily, too – but often don't. In a University of Nebraska Medical Center study that looked at almost 200 couples in which the man had had a heart attack or bypass surgery, it was found that in one in three households, *both* husbands and wives were overweight and they ate similar amounts of fat and salt. There were also similarities in their exercise levels as well as in their smoking histories. Indeed, women were twice as likely as their husbands to continue smoking eight weeks after their spouse's heart attack or heart surgery. *Many of the women did not even know their own blood cholesterol levels,* which, as we will explain, is an essential piece of knowledge for each of us.

Myth: A low-fat diet is the best thing for your heart.

Fact: The advice from the scientific community is no longer to keep dietary fat as low as possible. In fact, for some people, very low-fat diets can actually contribute to heart disease. The goal now is to keep only certain types of fat as low as possible. The limit for fats in general has been liberalized. Even up to 35 per cent of calories from fat is now considered acceptable (as long as it doesn't contribute to weight gain).

Myth: If you've been diagnosed with heart disease, you should not exercise.

Fact: If you've been diagnosed with heart disease, it is more important than ever to exercise. Gone are the weeks of bed rest for heart attack patients. Most are now encouraged to start moving their bodies again as soon as possible, even before they leave the hospital. Those with heart-related risk factors, such as high cholesterol, should be challenging their hearts to work harder with exercise, too.

Myth: Heart disease is an inevitable consequence of aging.

Fact: No, it's not. Yes, growing older puts you at higher heart disease risk. But risk is just that: risk. It's not a foregone conclusion, even for those with a family history of heart disease. There's much you can do in your everyday life to thwart 'fate'.

THE FEMALE HEART STEPS INTO THE SPOTLIGHT

The tide is shifting. As recently as 1958, paying attention to women's heart health was such an anomaly that heart disease researchers reporting on one of their studies noted it was 'the first time that any members of the "weaker sex" had participated in this work'. Today, that patronizing observation has been replaced with a policy handed down from the US federal government that half of all subjects in heart disease studies *must* be women in order for research funding to continue.

And the momentum is building. Only last year, both the American Heart Association (AHA) and the National Heart, Lung and Blood Institute in the US began campaigns to put women's heart disease risk front and centre. The AHA's campaign, a 'national call for women to take charge of their heart health and live stronger, longer lives' is called Go Red for Women. The National Heart, Lung and Blood Institute's programme is known as 'The Heart Truth: A National Awareness Campaign on Women and Heart Disease'. The AHA is the largest health advocacy organization focused on heart disease and stroke and the National Heart, Lung and Blood Institute is *the* major government agency focused on cardiovascular disease in the US. These changes represent an enormous step forwards.

The push to put the spotlight on women and heart disease comes not a moment too soon. It's especially pressing in light of all the recent negative findings on the effects of hormone replacement therapy (HRT). For years, women were told that HRT would protect them from heart disease and millions took it believing they were not only relieving menopausal symptoms and helping their bones but also taking care of their cardiovascular systems. Now, rigorously conducted research has concluded that there is a slight but significant increase in the risk for heart attacks with HRT – even within the first year of use.

With the HRT avenue of heart protection closed off, more than ever women need straightforward guidelines about how to take action to avoid their biggest killer – and how to take care of themselves should heart disease strike.

The good news: those guidelines are just coming together. The research on what women can do to protect themselves has reached the critical point at which it can be 'translated' for use, which is why we've written this book *now*.

NO MATTER WHERE YOU'RE STARTING FROM . . .

While you cannot change your genes or your age, there's much you *can* do to keep heart disease at bay or lessen its severity should it ever occur. That's true no matter what your starting fitness level, your current dietary habits or whether you're pre- or postmenopausal. Even if you've already been diagnosed with heart disease, you can dramatically reduce your risk that it will get worse. It's *never* too late to make a difference. You can start today with strategies that are entirely in your own control.

Strong Women, Strong Hearts lays it all out in terms you can understand – a complete programme that guides you through, step by step. There's nutrition, physical activity, weight control, relaxation and de-stressing techniques and much more. For instance, one of the most important components of living a heart-healthy lifestyle is diet, which is why we devote an entire chapter to that topic. The right eating pattern for heart health can reduce the risk for a future heart attack or stroke dramatically, yet it is one aspect of the heart protection issue that has become especially confusing. Is it low-fat and high-carbohydrate? High-protein and low-carbohydrate? What about soy – and oatmeal? Do they really lower cholesterol? Are red meat and eggs 'bad'? How much fish is right, especially given all the reports of contaminants in seafood?

To help you pull it all together, we distil the best research on the subject (some from our very own research groups and colleagues' laboratories) to offer a mix-and-match menu plan that allows you to choose the foods *you* prefer so that you'll stick with it. It works no matter what your eating style. There's no food *prescription*. While what you choose to eat can work as powerfully as medicine to keep down your heart disease risk, it should be *enjoyed*, not swallowed as a bitter pill.

Along with sound, flexible nutrition guidelines, we show you the latest in exercise to keep your heart primed as well as possible. It's not just aerobic exercises that count – walking, running, swimming, biking and so on. There's now convincing research that strength training is also very important for the conditioning of the entire cardiovascular system.

Even if you've never walked a mile or lifted a dumbbell in your life (an all-too-likely scenario since 76 per cent of women are sedentary), you'll be able to acclimatize yourself to this plan, outlined in the chapter on exercise. We give step-by-step instructions so that you can work up to a desirable fitness level *gradually.* You'll never be at a loss for what to do, how to measure your progress or how fast to go.

Those women who need to lose weight to lower their heart disease risk – or keep their weight from creeping up – will also get step-by-step instructions. We outline *the* ten strategies any woman should follow to lose weight healthily. You'll be amazed, even though you have to keep at it, at how much flexibility there is to a healthy weight-management plan *that works.*

While some chapters get at your heart through your eating habits and physical activity patterns, chapter 8 gets at your heart through your *soul.* Research has convincingly shown that your outlook in life – how angry you tend to get, how you channel that anger, how you connect with others, whether you are spiritually connected and so on – has a lot to do with the state of your heart. To that end, we offer strategies you can follow to get in touch with both yourself and those around you. That connectedness, in turn, will protect your heart from insidious damage that it can sustain from the stresses of day-to-day life.

There's also the manner in which you look out for yourself. Or do you? A lot of women tend to accommodate everyone else before themselves – at the expense of not only their own happiness but also their health. Women end up *dying* because they're so busy taking care of others that they don't stop to take care of themselves. The tendency not to challenge the status quo – leaving the doctor's office without answers to their questions, leaving the hospital without *really* having been taken care of, sacrificing their own needs in order not to 'make waves' – undercuts their ability to protect their hearts in very serious ways. In chapter 11, through one woman's life-and-death struggle to get her heart tended to, we advise you on how to *advocate* for yourself so that you get the help you need.

There is also a separate chapter on medications you might be prescribed to lower blood cholesterol or blood pressure and a chapter on procedures you may undergo to either help diagnose a heart problem or fix one – angiograms, bypasses, heart valve replacements and so on. We feel it is very important to have information on what you're going through or about to go through. That will allow you to ask the right questions as you get the care you need and in no small way relieve anxiety about medical therapies that you might otherwise be unfamiliar with. When anxiety is relieved, you will have more mental energy left to take the best possible care of yourself.

But long before you read through those chapters, you'll get a basic under-standing of how a heart – how a *woman's* heart – works, in chapter 2. The research underpinnings of all the lifestyle advice we have culled together will be explained early on, too, so you'll know *why* we're suggesting what we suggest.

You'll also be asked to answer several questions about yourself so you can ascertain your level of heart disease risk in the first place. Do you know your blood cholesterol level? Your level of physical fitness? Your blood pressure?

If not, you're not alone. Despite the advances, as an exercise physiologist (Miriam Nelson) and a heart disease researcher (Alice Lichtenstein), we are all too aware that many women's risk for cardiovascular illness is higher than they may realize. Indeed, it has meaning for us in a personal way, as it does for you. As women in middle age, we never want to be counted among the grim statistics ourselves. Nor do we want our daughters to be as they make their way through adolescence towards adulthood. The same sentiment goes for our older friends and relatives. We don't think *any* woman should be a heart disease target – which is why we've pulled together the latest research on women and heart disease and written this book.

We feel it's our *responsibility* to share the accumulated knowledge about how to stave off cardiovascular illness in women, just as it is now *your* responsibility to give voice to the issue and share your new found knowledge with others. The more women speak up – and make full use of the tools available – the greater the strides we can make.

It's time to put an end to the myth that heart disease wears only a shirt and tie, that women are immune from cardiovascular problems, that women don't need to take just as much care of their hearts as men do of theirs. By reading this book and following its guidelines, you're upending that myth and taking charge of your heart, in more ways than one.

CHAPTER 2

What Makes a Woman's Heart Unique?

◆

I told my doctor I had been having heartburn for three weeks and that my teeth ached. It was really more jaw pain, as if I were getting an electric shock in my jaw. She diagnosed gastric reflux and prescribed heartburn medi- cine. About thirty-six hours later, I had a major heart attack. I was 40.

— JUDY

When it comes to affairs of the heart, women definitely differ from men, whose heart disease often hits like a large truck rather than in the form of the more subtle symptoms women frequently experience. But to fully appreciate the differences, a general knowledge of how the heart works in all of us is needed.

HOW THE BEAT GOES ON

It's staggering when you stop to think about it. Almost from the time of conception until you draw your last breath, the heart beats *continuously* – dozens of times every single minute – in order to pump 4,300 gallons of blood each day to every organ and tissue in your body. By the time an 85-year-old woman dies, her heart has beaten an estimated 2,680,560,000 or 2.68 billion times.

The mechanism that keeps the heart pumping blood through the 100,000 miles of blood vessels in each of us (enough to circle the earth more than four times) is intricate, elegant and astounding almost beyond words.

The heart itself is made of muscle that squeezes in upon itself, or contracts, with every beat in order to push blood all the way down to your toes and up to your brain. The muscle is tightly bound in layers that form each of the heart's four chambers: the right atrium, the right ventricle, the left atrium and the left ventricle.

The Heart

LEFT ATRIUM

RIGHT ATRIUM

LEFT VENTRICLE

RIGHT VENTRICLE

Blood is pumped from the heart to the rest of the body directly from the left ventricle. When the layers of muscle making up the left ventricle contract, the resulting pressure is enough to push blood out of that chamber and then to all the body's arteries – blood vessels that carry blood *away* from the heart.

After the blood passes through all the arteries, it proceeds to the body's 10 billion capillaries. These tiny blood vessels are wide enough for only a single blood cell to pass at any one time. The advantage is that lots of very narrow blood tubules create an extremely large surface area through which oxygen and nutrients can be dropped off to all the cells that compose the various organs and other tissues making up the body. At the same time, carbon dioxide and other waste products are picked up.

From the capillaries, the blood flows to the veins – the vessels that carry blood *back* to the heart.

The Blood Pressure Connection

The pressure occurring at the peak of each heartbeat, when blood is pushed out to the entire body, is called *systolic pressure*, which is the first – and higher – number in a blood pressure reading.

Once the heart has pumped blood into the arteries and is between beats, blood pressure is at its lowest; no extra force is being exerted. That minimum pressure is called *diastolic pressure,* the second number in a blood pressure reading. Diastolic pressure, even when high, is always going to be a lower number than systolic pressure. That's because the pressure of blood against artery walls when the heart muscle first contracts is higher than the pressure in the tubes once the contraction is over and the blood being forced out of the heart has already done a fair amount of its travelling.

What numbers constitute high blood pressure, or hypertension (usually diagnosed with a cuff around your upper arm at routine doctor's visits)? Normal blood pressure? The cutoff points have recently been made more strict with evidence that lower blood pressure is more protective.

Blood pressure	Old classification	New classification (as of 2003)
<120/80 (mm/Hg)*	optimal	normal
120–129/80–84	normal	prehypertension
130–139/85–89	borderline	prehypertension
>140/90	hypertension	hypertension

* mm/Hg stands for millimetres of mercury, meaning the pressure is equivalent to the amount of pressure needed to drive a column of mercury up a tube of a specified width.

Once the blood returns to the heart, it enters through the right atrium (which houses the heart's natural pacemaker). From there it's pumped to the right ventricle. At that point, blood leaves the heart once again, this time for a short trip through the lungs. In the lungs, blood drops off carbon dioxide – a by-product of metabolism – and becomes replenished with oxygen that you've just breathed in. Then it flows into the heart's left atrium and from there to the left ventricle, where the whole process begins anew.

Take Your Resting Pulse

Your pulse, or heart rate, like your blood pressure, is an important indicator of how well your cardiovascular system is doing. Generally speaking, a low resting pulse – closer to, say, 55 beats per minute or lower rather than 70 or higher – indicates that your heart can pump more efficiently. That is, it can pump more blood with each beat and thereby transport plenty of oxygen and nutrients to all the cells of the body with less work.

How can you lower your pulse rate? Through regular exercise. Challenging the heart through aerobic exercise such as brisk walking, running, bicycling or swimming helps it to beat more efficiently. An elite athlete's resting heart rate can be as low as 30.

To find your resting pulse rate, first thing in the morning before you get out of bed, lightly put your fingers on an artery and count for 30 seconds. Then multiply by two since pulse rate is expressed in beats per minute. Most women can find an artery in either their wrist or their neck because the arteries in those spots are closest to the skin's surface. Beats are felt during the momentary increase in pressure that occurs as the heart muscle contracts. (To find your pulse rate during *exercise,* see the illustration and instructions on page 112.)

Of course, the many parts of this cycle are going on simultaneously. At the same time that deoxygenated blood is flowing through the veins back towards the heart, oxygen-rich blood is headed for the heart from the lungs. Blood is always leaving and approaching the heart at the same time.

When Something Goes Wrong

A system of valves within the heart makes sure blood doesn't flow in the wrong direction. For instance, the *tricuspid valve* separating the upper right chamber from the lower right chamber makes sure blood is always going from the atrium to the ventricle. Similarly, the *bicuspid,* or mitral, valve separates the upper and lower chambers of the left side of the heart. If the valve

The Cardiovascular System

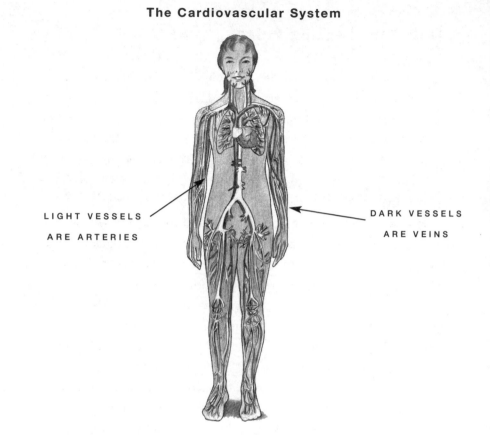

LIGHT VESSELS
ARE ARTERIES

DARK VESSELS
ARE VEINS

does not close completely and there's backward leakage, it's heard with a stethoscope as a *murmur*. Too much backward leakage and the valve may have to be repaired or even replaced.

But that kind of heart problem is very rare. It's not what most women need to be concerned about. The more common problem has to do with blood flow through the vessels that nourish the heart muscle. Consider that as blood is pumped away from the heart into arteries that bring it to all the organs and tissues of the body, it is also pumped into arteries that nourish the heart muscle itself. After all, the heart muscle, like all other body tissues, needs to have a constant supply of oxygen and nutrients delivered by the blood. And that blood does not come directly from the heart's four chambers but, as with any other organ, from arteries. These arteries are on the outer surface of the heart.

The arteries that bring blood to the heart muscle are referred to as coronary arteries. If any of them become narrowed or partly blocked, not enough oxygen will reach the heart muscle, interfering with function. This happens when cholesterol-rich plaque builds up in them, impeding blood flow and it's called *coronary heart disease.* (A more general term for blocked arteries is *atherosclerosis,* from the Greek *athero* – gruel or paste – and *sclerosis* – hardness.)

But heart disease is not necessarily just a 'plumbing' problem. Blood flow can also be impeded as an indirect result of inflammation. When an atherosclerotic artery becomes inflamed, plaque becomes unstable and can rupture, precipitating the formation of a blood clot – and a subsequent heart attack or stroke.

The Progression of Atherosclerosis
The left vessel is relatively free of plaque. The right vessel has advanced plaque and is much more likely to result in blocked blood flow.

Barring an out-and-out coronary event, the heart muscle's blood oxygen deprivation may be felt as *angina* – chest pain or discomfort, perhaps accompanied by pain in the shoulders, arms, neck, jaw or back. Sometimes angina may be felt on exertion, for example, while hurrying to catch a plane, carrying groceries in from the car or vacuuming. In such cases, it is known as stable angina. More concerning is unstable angina. The symptoms occur at rest, which suggests that even without exertion, not enough oxygen is getting to the heart muscle. Recently, it has become apparent that in women in particular, angina may also manifest itself simply as fatigue or feeling 'not quite right'.

Angina and heart attacks occur on a continuum. If the plaque buildup sufficiently narrows a coronary artery, or if even a small amount of plaque made unstable by inflammation causes the formation of a blood clot, most or all blood flow will be cut off and a heart attack, or *myocardial infarction,* can occur. Blood clots can form anywhere in the body, especially if the blood vessels are inflamed and then travel to – and get stuck in – a coronary artery or they can form right in a coronary artery itself, causing the abrupt cessation of blood flow. Of course, the more narrowed an artery becomes by plaque, or the more inflammation that is present, the more likely that a clot will block off blood flow.

How Does Plaque Form?

Plaque, which narrows arteries and contributes to the formation of clots, both of which can lead to heart attacks, is made primarily of cholesterol. The majority of cholesterol comes straight from the blood circulating through the body, either directly or indirectly from what is called 'bad' LDL-cholesterol, which is why it's so important to keep down LDL-cholesterol levels in the blood.

One way cholesterol is prevented from accumulating in arteries has to do with 'good' HDL-cholesterol. How HDL-cholesterol works is complicated, but to oversimplify for a moment, consider that both LDL- and HDL-cholesterol are made from cholesterol and protein. However, the kind of protein in each is different. The protein that is part of LDL-cholesterol causes it to be deposited as plaque on blood vessel walls. The protein that helps make up HDL-cholesterol, on the other hand, enables cholesterol to be picked up from blood vessel walls and carried to the liver via a process called *reverse cholesterol transport.*

The liver, in turn, rids the body of cholesterol in a number of ways. For instance, it can use the cholesterol to make bile acids, which are necessary for digestion. Or it can secrete cholesterol directly into the small intestine to be eliminated from the body.

When Your Brain *Doesn't Get Enough Blood*

The same principle that applies to arteries nourishing the heart also applies to narrowing of the carotid (kah-ROT-id) arteries, the main arteries in the neck that supply blood to the brain. Such blockage is called *carotid artery stenosis* and the result in this case can be a brain attack, more commonly known as a stroke.

There are actually two kinds of stroke. About 80 per cent are ischemic strokes, in which a clot lodges in either the carotid artery or a smaller artery branching out from it. The result is that part of the brain does not get adequate blood; hence, there's an inadequate supply of oxygen, which can kill brain cells. How such a stroke plays out is highly variable, depending on which part of the brain is affected, how large the affected brain region is and for how long the vessel is blocked. Some people have TIAs, or transient ischemic attacks – greatly diminished blood flow that lasts only a couple of minutes and has no long-term effects (although people who have them are at much higher risk for more serious strokes later). At the other extreme are massive ischemic strokes, which cause paralysis, difficulty speaking and potentially death.

The other 20 per cent of strokes are haemorrhagic strokes – haemorrhaging or bleeding, into the brain from one of the brain's blood vessels. This type also leads to variable consequences, depending on the brain region affected and the severity of the bleeding. High blood pressure is a major risk factor for haemorrhagic stroke.

Other possible problems (which, unlike blocked arteries, are not always directly affected by lifestyle) include aneurysms, arrhythmias, atrial fibrillation, congestive heart failure and peripheral vascular disease. For definitions, consult the glossary.

HEART DISEASE'S FEMININE TOUCH

With men, often the first sign of heart disease is a heart attack itself or at least a distinct tightening or squeezing in the chest upon exertion. Women's first warning signs are often much more subtle: shortness of breath or fatigue when engaging in activities that used to be easy or even a feeling of mild indigestion. Sometimes there's *diffuse* chest pain. But in one study of 515 women who had had heart attacks, 43 per cent said they never experienced any chest discomfort whatsoever; 95 per cent, on the other hand, experienced relatively vague symptoms such as fatigue and sleeplessness up to a month before they were struck.

The male–female differences go deeper than just the symptoms. There are differences in the blood vessels themselves. Women's arteries tend to be smaller than men's. Therefore, if a woman has to undergo bypass surgery, which is a rerouting of blood via insertion of a healthy blood vessel to bypass one that is blocked or nearly blocked, the operation is more difficult and more risky. Perhaps that's one of the reasons that in a review of more than 300,000 people undergoing bypass surgery, the death rate was higher in women.

Women's Hearts React Differently to Emotions

It's not just physical differences that make women's hearts different from men's. Feelings play out differently, too. As you may have heard and could probably intuit even if you haven't, men with type-A personalities are more likely than other men to die after a heart attack, at least according to preliminary research. The stress, anger and impatience apparently do them in. What's not so commonly known is that women appear more likely to die after a heart attack if they *don't* show their anger and instead react slowly to negative events, suppressing unpleasant emotions such as agitation during stressful times. In the well-known Framingham Heart Study in the US, women who reported suppressing their anger experienced the highest rate of first heart attacks.

We suspect that there must be a happy middle ground – not flying off the handle at every opportunity but not keeping everything bottled up inside, either.

Isolation may be bad for women's hearts as well. In primate research, being socially isolated and having limited freedom of movement was correlated with greater heart disease among females. And female monkeys housed alone have been found to suffer more extensive atherosclerosis than their counterparts housed in social groups.

But what makes women's hearts *most* unlike men's is not their heart disease symptoms, nor the apparatus that makes up their cardiovascular systems, nor the way their hearts react to emotional stress or social situations. It's the way their hearts are *perceived* – both by doctors and by women themselves.

WOMEN'S HEARTS UNDER-ATTENDED BY THE MEDICAL COMMUNITY

Bypass surgery may be trickier to perform on women's narrower arteries, but an even bigger problem is that fewer women who need bypasses ever get them. There continues to linger a perception on the part of the health care community that heart disease is a man's illness. In one Canadian study of more than 30,000 people who had had either a heart attack or unstable angina, women were 30 per cent less likely than men to undergo revascularization – procedures to open up blocked blood vessels. In fact, women undergo intensive treatment for heart disease much less frequently than men with symptoms of the same severity. Sometimes a man with *less* severe symptoms than a woman will still be more likely to get more intensive treatment. When researchers at the Tufts–New England Medical Center conducted a study of 889 patients with acute angina, they found that only 2 per cent were mistakenly discharged from hospital emergency departments around the country. But the percentage for women under age 55 was much greater. They were *seven* times more likely not to be admitted straight from casualty than were people in other groups.

Women's seemingly vague symptoms continue not to be recognized as frequently as men's for the heart attacks they can turn out to be. Even the way doctors manage chest pain itself has been shown to be influenced by the gender of the patient. As you'll see in a later chapter, in some cases a woman's symptoms have to be extreme before her heart disease is fully recognized for what it is.

When women *are* finally treated for cardiovascular problems, it's often very late in their disease development and therefore less likely to be helpful. For instance, women who do undergo bypass surgery typically are sicker and older than their male counterparts. Due to late detection and intervention, their heart disease is more advanced and therefore more severe.

It's not just *treatment* that's lacking for women. So are *evaluation* and diagnostic procedures. Women who have had a heart attack are less likely than male heart attack patients to undergo cardiac catheterization, a procedure that analyzes blood flow in the arteries leading to the heart in order to ascertain the location and extent of the damage. Women doctors prescribe the test to their female patients just as infrequently as male doctors do, according to a study that looked at the records of 104,000 US Medicare heart patients.

Women are also less likely to undergo the standard treadmill test that helps ascertain heart disease risk. Think about it: when the treadmill test comes to mind, we tend to envision a man huffing and puffing to exhaustion.

But a woman's level of fitness, measured by a standardized treadmill exercise test, might be even more predictive of whether she'll die than a man is. In a 2003 study conducted at Chicago's Rush Institute, researchers followed 5,700 women who had had their exercise capacity assessed on treadmills. Eight years later, those who were not able to work up to walking at least 2.5 miles per hour on an incline with a 12 per cent gradient (equivalent to a very steep hill) were almost twice as likely to die as those who could. Women who couldn't progress even to 1.7 miles an hour on a 10 per cent incline (still a rather steep hill) were three times as likely to die during that eight-year span. **The results showed physical fitness to be an even more important predictor of death for women than for men – by twofold.** For this reason, we have included a physical fitness test in the next chapter to help you assess your heart disease risk.

WOMEN'S HEARTS UNDER-ATTENDED BY WOMEN THEMSELVES

If glossing over the state of women's hearts by the medical community isn't enough, women themselves often give their hearts short shrift. In fact, one of the reasons women die more often than men following a heart attack is that they wait longer to go to the hospital when they're having one; hence, more heart muscle has already died by the time they receive treatment.

Women are inclined to ignore or downplay red flags because they don't *expect* to get heart disease, even though it's their number-one killer. They misinterpret their own less-than-clear-cut symptoms. Indeed, while more than *ten times* as many women die of cardiovascular disease than of breast cancer, women think their risk of dying from heart disease is only twice the risk of dying from breast cancer, according to one survey. Of even greater concern, the same survey indicates that only 7 per cent of women consider heart disease their greatest problem, whereas 34 per cent cite breast cancer.

Can Your Daily Routine Provide a Hint About Your Heart Disease Risk?

Men often don't get clues that a heart attack is in the offing. They feel absolutely fine one moment and are laid low the next. Women have an advantage in that regard. If a woman has to slow down to get tasks done, if she gets winded doing something that she used to be able to do with ease, if she simply has to stop doing something that's very important to her, it can be a sign of heart disease or even an impending heart attack. And such early warning signs – if recognized – can allow a woman to get help before a lot of damage is done.

Unfortunately, doctors don't tend to ask questions about daily routine when they assess patients for heart disease. They talk about more intense kinds of physical activity, like brisk walking or swimming. Also, a doctor may ask, 'Are you having chest pains?' But that question can be misleading. A woman may answer no simply because she has stopped doing something, or started doing it more slowly, in order to avoid chest pains. At the same time, a doctor may *not* ask about symptoms that could be very telling, such as fatigue or a vague feeling of nausea.

To keep from falling through the cracks before heart disease has gone too far, all women should periodically ask themselves a series of questions about their ability to perform routine activities. For instance, many women, over time, have to modify the way they do things like carry laundry up the stairs or change the sheets. (Changing bed linens, which research has shown can take a fair amount of energy, has been marked as the household task most commonly done differently because of heart disease symptoms. Women stop for rests more or do the work more slowly.) So one of the questions should be:

Can I handle housework without difficulty or has it become more difficult? Do I have to rest in the middle of a chore that I used to be able to sail through without taking breaks?

Other potential questions:

- Have I stopped doing outside work and gardening as rigorously as I used to?
- Have I developed a habit of letting things accumulate at the bottom of the stairs so I only have to make one trip upstairs each day?
- Do I now check in my bags before boarding a flight because it has become too hard to walk through the airport with them?
- Has it got harder for me to carry things in from the car?

If the answers to these and other questions related to your daily habits are yes, it does not necessarily mean you have heart disease. There are lots of reasons a woman might not be able to do something as well as she used to: arthritis pain, for instance, or back trouble or just plain old slowing down with aging. But a decline in ability to do chores that are very important to you or that you used to complete as a matter of course should serve as a signal that it's time to make a doctor's appointment.

TURNING THE TIDE

Lack of attention to the possibility of heart disease also means lack of attention to prevention. When you think of a heart attack victim, you probably think of an overweight man, perhaps a smoker, who doesn't get any exercise and doesn't watch what he eats. But take a look at the numbers. An estimated 34 per cent of all women in the US and UK are overweight and another 30 per cent in the US (19 per cent in the UK) are obese. Twenty-five per cent of American women report that they do no regular physical activity. (That number goes up as women age.) Twenty-two million American women smoke. The prevalence of high blood pressure, another major heart disease risk factor, is *rising* in women but not in men – no doubt at least in part because women are getting heavier. In other words, women fit the heart attack profile, too.

The silver lining in all this is that women can lower their heart disease risk

– both by living more healthily and by becoming more attuned to possible signs of heart trouble. Armed with that greater awareness, a woman is in a much better position to work together with her doctor both to avoid heart disease and, if need be, to identify it in its early stages so that it can be attended to before any major damage is done. In the chapters that follow, you'll learn how.

CHAPTER 3

Take the Test to Learn Your Risk

◆

I suspected high blood pressure was coming. My sister, who is twelve years younger than I am, has had high blood pressure since she was in her thirties. And both my mother and father have it. I wasn't too concerned about my cholesterol, however. It had always been fine. In fact, I had got a little cocky about it, not being as careful about eating healthily and all that (although I was still thin). But when my doctor finally checked it again after several years, it had gone way up.

— ANNE

How likely are you to suffer a heart attack, stroke or other coronary 'event' in the next ten years? Do you have a 10 per cent chance? Twenty per cent? Greater than 20 per cent?

These are not theoretical questions. Every single woman, particularly by age 40, should know her risk for developing cardiovascular disease so that she can develop an appropriate game plan for preventing it. There's an imperative for preventing that first heart attack, stroke or other coronary complication. The rate of first 'events' that are disabling, and even fatal, is very high. Fifty per cent of people having a heart attack die before they ever get to the hospital.

Maybe you assume you're at low risk and therefore don't need to be concerned. But almost 40 per cent of women, as well as men, in the United States are at *moderate* risk, meaning they have an elevated chance of experiencing a heart attack or other cardiovascular-related calamity that could prove deadly. They need to take some specific steps to protect themselves. Unfortunately, many of them – perhaps the majority – don't know it, because they don't know how to assess their own risk for heart disease or because they have never been concerned about it.

Granted, in some cases their doctors may know it, assigning them a risk score periodically. But *you* should be aware of it, too. One reason is that the better informed you are, the more committed you'll be to making the changes necessary to lower your chances of having a heart attack or stroke. At least as important, a lot of people fall through cracks in the medical system. Either they aren't treated aggressively enough or they're treated *too* aggressively, being slapped with a drug prescription before they've had a chance to see if changes in diet and physical activity patterns alone are enough to improve heart health. Keeping apprised of your risk level will help you to work *with* your doctor by allowing you to keep track of whether you're following the *right* plan for protecting your heart.

PUTTING A NUMBER TO IT

Exactly how do you quantify your heart disease risk? There's a scoring system put out by the US National Heart, Lung and Blood Institute that's often used as an initial screening tool. Fortunately, it's extremely easy to tally up, requiring that you answer only five questions about yourself (other than your gender): your age, total blood cholesterol, smoking status, HDL-cholesterol level ('good' cholesterol) and systolic blood pressure (that first number in a blood pressure reading).

Obviously, you'll need to get a couple of these answers during a physical at your doctor's surgery. If you've had a physical within the last two years that also included blood work and a blood pressure reading, you can call the doctor's surgery for the numbers. If more time than that has gone by, you should still call the doctor's surgery – to make an appointment. (Before you read on, write a note to yourself in the margin of this page or on a slip of paper as a reminder to phone your doctor's surgery, if necessary.)

The doctor will draw blood to measure your total and HDL-cholesterol and, in many cases, your LDL-cholesterol level as well. If the numbers are outside the desirable range, you will probably be asked to come back and have blood drawn after an overnight fast to confirm the reading. At that time, the doctor will also tell the lab to check your LDL-cholesterol (if it wasn't previously measured) and your blood triglyceride level, which can be correctly determined only after a fast. (See the box on page 32 for more on triglycerides.)

You'll see below that each answer to the five questions is assigned a certain value. Add the total points for your five answers, then match the sum to your ten-year risk. As the chart makes clear, if your point total falls below 20, your coronary heart disease risk is below 10 per cent, which means it's low. If your point total runs between 20 and 22, your coronary heart disease risk is between 10 and 20 per cent, which means it's moderate. And a score of 23 or higher means your chance of suffering from heart disease or any of its complications over the next ten years is greater than 20 per cent – high. (*Your risk is automatically considered greater than 20 per cent if you already have heart disease or diabetes, no matter what your score on these five questions.*)

1. Age	Points	Age	Points
20–34	-7	55–59	8
35–39	-3	60–64	10
40–44	0	65–69	12
45–49	3	70–74	14
50–54	6	75 and up	16

2. Total Cholesterol	Age				
(milligrams per decilitre of blood)	20–39	40–49	50–59	60–69	70–79
	Points				
Less than 160	0	0	0	0	0
160–199	4	3	2	1	1
200–239	8	6	4	2	1
240–279	11	8	5	3	2
At or greater than 280	13	10	7	4	2

3. Smoking History	Age				
	20–39	40–49	50–59	60–69	70–79
	Points				
Nonsmoker	0	0	0	0	0
Smoker	9	7	4	2	1

4. HDL-Cholesterol

(milligrams per decilitre of blood)	Points
60 or above	-1
50–59	0
40–49	1
Less than 40	2

5. Systolic Blood Pressure	If Untreated	If Treated
Less than 120	0	0
120–129	1	3
130–139	2	4
140–159	3	5
At least 160	4	6

YOUR TOTAL POINTS: _____

Point Total	Your Ten–Year Risk	
	(% chance of experiencing a heart attack)	
Less than 9	Less than 1%	Low Risk
9–12	1	Low Risk
13–14	2	Low Risk
15	3	Low Risk

Point Total	Your Ten–Year Risk (% chance of experiencing a heart attack)	
16	4	Low Risk
17	5	Low Risk
18	6	Low Risk
19	8	Low Risk
20	11	Moderate Risk
21	14	Moderate Risk
22	17	Moderate Risk
23	22	High Risk
24	27	High Risk
25 or more	At least 30%	High Risk

How high your risk is dictates just how aggressive you should be in your heart disease prevention efforts. For instance, if it's less than 10 per cent, and therefore low, there's probably not much you need to alter in your current lifestyle to keep heart disease at bay. But if your chance of suffering a heart attack or related problem over the next ten years is at least 20 per cent, or high, you'll need to take more intensive measures to get it down, by making more of an effort to lose some excess weight, if need be, in addition to eating a more healthy diet in general and exercising appropriately. In addition, your doctor will probably start you on a drug regimen. For someone at high risk, lifestyle and medications together can be a powerful deterrent of cardiovascular events.

If you're at moderate risk for having a heart attack or a related event in the next ten years, 10 to 20 per cent, the intensity of your lifestyle efforts and whether you should take a drug will be a judgement call.

What About LDL-Cholesterol?

Your level of LDL-cholesterol presently isn't used to calculate your ten-year heart disease risk, but your risk score dictates, in part, what your LDL-cholesterol level should be. Indeed, there may be nothing more important you can do than to keep down your LDL-cholesterol.

To determine the LDL-cholesterol that is right for you, you also need to tally how many risk factors you have; the more you have, the higher your risk. The risk factors that are especially applicable to *women* (we know you have already factored in some of them):

- Cigarette smoking
- High blood pressure (at or greater than 140/90 without medication)
- Low HDL-cholesterol (less than 50 mg/dl)
- Family history of premature heart disease (under age 65 in a female first-degree relative and under age 55 in a male first-degree relative)
- Age (at least 55)

People at low risk for heart disease, as indicated by your point score and your number of risk factors, are considered healthier with higher levels of LDL-cholesterol in their blood than people at moderate or high risk. Simply put, they have more room for manoeuvre for higher LDL-cholesterol levels.

Level of Risk (from pages 27–28)	LDL-Cholesterol Goal (milligrams per decilitre of blood)
10-year risk below 10% + 0–1 risk factor	160 or lower
10-year risk below 10% + 2 or more risk factors	130 or lower
10-year risk of 10–20% + 2 or more risk factors	130 or lower (Your doctor may set an LDL goal closer to 100)
10-year risk of 20% or higher	100 or lower (Your doctor may set an LDL goal closer to 70)

Note: You can subtract one risk factor from the total if your HDL-cholesterol is above 60 mg/dl.

Do You Have Metabolic Syndrome?

While keeping LDL-cholesterol appropriately low is the most critical step for warding off a heart attack or other cardiovascular event, it's also important to determine whether you have something called *metabolic syndrome* – and to get treatment if you do. Metabolic syndrome in itself raises the chances of heart disease, independently of LDL-cholesterol levels.

How do you determine whether you have metabolic syndrome? You can't *feel* it; there are no symptoms. Rather, it's a cluster of risk factors. If, with your doctor, you determine that you have at least three out of the following risk factors, you've got it.

- Abdominal obesity (waist circumference greater than 35 inches)*
- High triglycerides (at least 150 milligrams per decilitre of blood)
- Low HDL-cholesterol (less than 50 milligrams per decilitre of blood)*
- High blood pressure (at least 130/85)
- High blood sugar, or fasting glucose, which is a precursor to diabetes (at least 110 milligrams per decilitre of blood)

Management of metabolic syndrome, which occurs as frequently in postmenopausal women as in men, includes a combination of weight loss, dietary modification and increased physical activity and, in some cases, medications. These approaches will also reduce LDL-cholesterol in someone who has high levels.

People with metabolic syndrome must not go on a very low-fat diet, which could actually exacerbate the condition by increasing triglyceride levels, as we will explain shortly.

The numbers apply specifically to women.

Other Important Factors to Consider

You may be wondering why some other important numbers aren't part of the US National Heart, Lung and Blood Institute's scoring system: your weight, for instance, or the amount of time you spend in moderately vigorous physical activity. Part of the reason is that this self-assessment measures your *primary* risk factors for heart disease. For example, your weight certainly influences your risk, but it's *secondary*. That is, excess weight is a risk factor because it tends to increase primary risk factors such as blood cholesterol, blood pressure and elevated blood sugar. Indeed, women who are even only a little bit overweight can be at as much as a sevenfold increased risk for heart disease compared to their thinner counterparts, according to findings from Harvard's Nurses' Health Study. Still, excess weight in and of itself does not increase your chances of having a heart attack or stroke. It's the high cholesterol, hypertension and high blood sugar levels that do that.

There are other things that influence risk secondarily that are also worth considering. For instance, both the Iowa Women's Study and the Nurses' Health Study, which combined follow some 150,000 women, have reported that women who eat diets with more daily servings of whole grains, fruits and vegetables than other women are at decreased risk for developing heart disease. It's hard to tease out exactly how that dietary pattern works. We do know that whole grains and produce contain fibre, which can play a role in lowering blood cholesterol. Diets that are high in fibre also tend to be relatively low in calories. Therefore, this kind of eating pattern can help keep down weight. It also helps ward off diabetes, which is a very big heart disease risk in itself, especially in women. Finally, healthy diets rich in vegetables, fruits and whole grains leave less room for foods like pastries, ice cream, biscuits, sweets and fatty cuts of meat, all of which can negatively influence blood cholesterol and thereby raise heart disease risk.

Considering Triglycerides

One of the most hotly debated questions in the cardiovascular field is how important the level of triglycerides in your blood is for estimating your heart disease risk. One study published several years ago in the *Archives of Internal Medicine* (the American Medical Association's journal) found that triglyceride levels in women (but not in men) were useful for estimating heart disease risk. But the number of women observed was too small to draw any conclusions with confidence and the issue is not straightforward in the first place.

One of the reasons it's not at all clear whether high triglyceride levels provide additional information about disease risk is that in the majority of cases, when triglycerides are high, HDL-cholesterol is low and vice versa. Even more to the point for women actively trying to lower their chance for heart disease is that the approach to lowering high triglyceride levels overlaps with that for raising HDL-cholesterol levels – lose excess weight and increase physical activity.

If you're overweight and lose more than 10 per cent of your body weight, you may be able to lower your triglycerides by as much as 30 to 40 per cent at the same time that you raise HDL-cholesterol. And there is preliminary evidence that if you become more physically active, you can lower triglycerides by as much as 10 per cent and again, raise HDL-cholesterol.

Put another way, screening for triglycerides may be something of a moot point. You should already be doing what it takes to keep those levels down. The only thing some women with high triglycerides may be advised to do in addition to taking the other lifestyle steps is cut down *a little* on carbohydrates (fewer cakes, biscuits, pasta and white bread) and replace the lost calories with *a little* unsaturated fat, such as vegetable oil or the fat in fish. A very low-fat diet can raise triglycerides dramatically in some women.

Triglyceride Categories (which must be assessed via a blood test
taken after an overnight fast)

Normal: less than 150 (milligrams per decilitre
                             of blood)
Borderline high: 150–199
High: 200–499
Very high: 500 or more

THE FITNESS FACTOR

As far as physical activity level, a sedentary lifestyle is considered an important risk factor for heart disease. It directly influences a woman's chances of having a heart attack or stroke down the line. One reason it's not part of the risk scoring system is that in certain ways, it's hard to measure exactly the degree to which fitness impacts heart disease risk. We know that being active reduces blood pressure and blood glucose, improves circulation and HDL-cholesterol levels and helps promote weight control, for instance, but not all the connections on a biological level have been fully researched. Still, it has become clear that physical inactivity, in conjunction with a poor diet, is about to eclipse tobacco as the leading cause of death in the US.

For that reason we feel it's very important for women to take a fitness assessment in addition to the assessment at the beginning of this chapter. It will give you at least some indication of whether your current fitness level is decreasing your heart disease risk or contributing to it. You can return to this assessment after the physical activity programme outlined in chapter 6 becomes a habit. Every three months is reasonable for monitoring your progress. You may be surprised at the positive changes.

How Fit Are You?

If you can comfortably walk a mile, take this simple test to estimate your aerobic fitness: walk for 12 minutes as fast as you can. Over the coming weeks and months, repeat the test to track your fitness progress.

This assessment tool was developed by colleagues of ours at the Cooper Institute in Dallas. They tested hundreds of women (and men) and came up with the chart on page 35, which has been shown to compare very well for accuracy to the numbers generated by more technical physical fitness assessment procedures.

Take the Cooper Test

Step 1: Take the Par-Q questionnaire on page 104 to see if you need to check with your doctor before taking the test.

Step 2: Find a local track you have permission to use, such as at a high school, college or community centre, and find out how many laps equal a mile.

Step 3: Select a day when the weather is good. Dress in comfortable clothes and athletic shoes. Bring along a stopwatch – or a watch with big hands and an easy-to-read face – plus a pencil and paper.

Step 4: Before the test, warm up for five minutes by walking at a moderate pace.

Step 5: Start the stopwatch and walk as fast as you can *for 12 minutes.* If you regularly run or jog, you may do so for all or part of the test.

Step 6: Note the number of laps around the track you complete, including any partial distance you cover during the final lap, before the 12 minutes are up.

Step 7: Slow your pace and cool down by walking slowly for five minutes.

Step 8: Write down the number of times you went around the track, including the partial distance of the final lap. Calculate the distance that you covered. Check the chart to determine your fitness level.

	Cooper Twelve-Minute Walking/Running Test *Distance Covered (in Miles) in Twelve Minutes*					
FITNESS CATEGORY	**AGE**					
	13–19	**20–29**	**30–39**	**40–49**	**50–59**	**60+**
Superior	>1.52	>1.46	>1.40	>1.35	>1.31	>1.19
Excellent	1.44–1.51	1.35–1.45	1.30–1.39	1.25–1.35	1.19–1.30	1.10–1.18
Good	1.30–1.43	1.23–1.34	1.19–1.29	1.12–1.24	1.06–1.18	.99–1.09
Fair	1.19–1.29	1.12–1.22	1.06–1.18	.99–1.11	.94–1.05	.87–.98
Poor	1.00–1.18	.96–1.11	.95–1.05	.88–.98	.84–.93	.78–.86
Very Poor	<1.0	<.96	<.94	<.88	<.84	<.78

Laps covered: _____

Distance in miles: _____

Your age: _____

Determine your fitness level: _____

If you fall into the 'Excellent' or 'Superior' category, congratulate yourself; fitness-wise, you are at a relatively low risk for heart disease. That doesn't mean that you don't need to exercise (or control and improve other risk factors). It means you have a good fitness foundation from which to proceed. If you are in the 'Good' category, there is room for improvement and your health will benefit if you become more fit. If you score 'Fair' or lower, your heart is incontrovertibly being compromised by your fitness level. The good news is that by following the *Strong Women, Strong Hearts* exercise programme, outlined in chapter 6, your fitness level will soar – and so will your heart health.

EMERGING RISK FACTORS

The nature of heart disease research is such that new risk factors are being discovered all the time. It is not yet clear how powerfully they influence the chances of having a heart attack or stroke, but scientists are busy determining whether doctors should be ordering lab tests for some of them. Here's a rundown.

High-Sensitivity C-Reactive Protein

If you're at moderate risk for heart disease – you scored a 10 to 20 per cent chance of suffering a cardiovascular event in the next ten years – you should talk to your doctor about whether it's advisable to get a test for what's known as high-sensitivity C-reactive protein, or CRP. The CRP test checks for inflammation in the body, arteries included. While a high level of cholesterol means there is probably a buildup of plaque in the arteries that impedes the flow of blood (at least in part), a high CRP score means there's a chance that there's a lot of *inflammation* in the arteries. And that inflammation, which can be brought on by such factors as injury to blood vessel walls, cigarette smoking and high blood pressure, can cause any of the plaque present to potentially rupture – triggering clots that might bring on a heart attack or stroke.

The test is not advised for people at low risk for heart disease because a high number wouldn't alter the lifestyle recommendations. A CRP test also isn't recommended for people at high risk because they should already be receiving aggressive treatment – making very intensive efforts with their diet and physical activity patterns and, if necessary, taking drugs to bring down their cholesterol level or treat other risk factors. But for patients at moderate risk for whom doctors are undecided about prescribing drugs, the outcome of the CRP test could help them make up their minds.

Note: While you should definitely have your CRP tested if your doctor recommends it, some of the latest reports question its value in predicting heart disease risk. One reason is that because the test signifies inflammation anywhere in the body, not just the arteries, a high value could be a false alarm. Even someone with a minor cold or a flare-up due to an infection can have an elevated level. In addition, there is some evidence that the test as a whole doesn't hold up nearly as strongly as a predictive measure for heart disease in women as in men. Thus, CRP levels should be interpreted very cautiously.

Homocysteine

Some evidence suggests that high blood levels of homocysteine (ho-mo-CIS-teen), a metabolic product of an amino acid found in proteins, is a marker for heart disease. Homocysteine builds up not because someone eats too much protein but for a variety of other reasons, including a low intake of certain B vitamins.

Researchers suspect that excess homocysteine may damage the lining of blood vessels or trigger the growth of cells that help form fatty deposits, namely plaque, on artery walls. It may also accelerate artery damage by encouraging the breakdown of LDL-cholesterol within plaque, adding to damage that results in the arteries becoming harder and less supple.

But it's not proven. It may be that homocysteine doesn't *cause* artery damage but, rather, is the *result* of it. If that's the case, lowering homocysteine in the blood won't actually reduce the risk for developing heart disease. Scientists are still working out cause and effect.

Given the uncertainties, doctors are divided on whether they should test for homocysteine routinely. On the plus side, the test is relatively inexpensive, usually running somewhere between £15 and £25. On the minus side, it's another number that can cause anxiety when, in fact, it may not have any predictive value. (A number above 12 – micromoles per litre of blood – is generally considered high.)

The good news is that, for most people, reducing homocysteine levels in the blood is not difficult. Colleagues of ours at Tufts have helped demonstrate that you just have to make sure to eat enough of the following three B vitamins: folate, B_6 and B_{12}. Our eating plan in chapter 5 will ensure that you do.

Small, Dense LDL

It's not just knowing how much LDL-cholesterol you have that's important. It's also knowing the *size* of the LDL particles, some researchers believe. The smaller the LDL particles, the denser they are and the heavier for their size.

That means they are most likely to remain in your bloodstream and eventually be taken up by cells that add to plaque more readily than large, 'puffy' LDL particles.

It's not clear who are the best candidates for small dense LDL screening. Furthermore, the test is expensive (about £120), few health insurance companies will reimburse for it and few laboratories can do it in-house. Just as important, the medical community is not convinced that it should be a standard part of anyone's diagnostic care. More to the point, your doctor most likely would not use the information to treat you differently than if she/he did not have the information. It's still too new, particularly given the fact that we don't yet know how prominently small dense LDL figures in heart disease risk in the majority of women. Additionally, it is not clear *how* to shift the balance from small dense to large LDL. Any recommendation would be the same as what would be given to reduce elevated LDL-cholesterol levels.

ApoE4

Every single person has a gene called apoE on chromosome number 19. About 15 per cent of the population has a form of that gene, or mutation, called apoE4 (as opposed to the most common form, apoE3, or a rarer form, apoE2), which makes them particularly prone to high blood cholesterol if they eat a high-fat diet – and puts them at higher risk of developing heart disease. The flip side is that individuals with the apoE4 mutation are more likely to respond to changes in their diets.

The reality is, genetic testing isn't yet part of routine medical exams; it would be too expensive at this point to do on a patient-by-patient basis. So very few people know which form of the apoE gene they have. But not too many years down the line, it is expected that efficient, inexpensive ways to sequence people's genes will be developed, which will allow doctors (and their patients!) to know who has to be more careful about limiting saturated fat in the diet, keeping down their weight and so on.

Lipoprotein Associated Phospholipase A2 (Lp-PLA2)

An enzyme known as Lp-PLA2 is released by white blood cells in response to inflammation. It travels through the bloodstream by piggybacking onto LDL particles, causing the release of material from the particles that can make plaque on the artery walls more likely to rupture and trigger a blood clot that can lead to a heart attack.

Screening for Lp-PLA2 might be useful as a predictor of heart disease risk in people with low LDL levels. Theoretically, if you have low LDL-cholesterol levels, you're at low heart disease risk, but there are plenty of people with low LDL who have heart attacks. It has been observed that a number of them have relatively high concentrations of Lp-PLA2. The thinking is that the more of that enzyme you have, the more likely that even a small amount of LDL-cholesterol in your bloodstream can both trigger plaque growth and the likelihood that the plaque will rupture, causing the formation of an obstructing clot.

The US Food and Drug Administration formally approved a lab test for Lp-PLA2 in July 2003. But at this point, whether to screen for the substance or not is at the doctor's discretion. There are no formal recommendations because the value of the screen has yet to be adequately evaluated.

Myeloperoxidase (MPO)

Emerging research suggests that this protein works in similar fashion to Lp-PLA2. It's released in response to inflammation and its presence has been related to plaque instability, meaning that it is more likely to form a life-threatening clot. But whereas Lp-PLA2 works through LDL-cholesterol particles that then influence plaque, MPO acts more directly on the plaque itself. Screening of MPO has yet to be approved in the US by the Food and Drug Administration.

RISK IS A MOVING TARGET

Knowing your risk for heart disease is critical not only because it lets you know how high your chances are for developing heart disease. As we said earlier, it's also an excellent motivator for making the lifestyle changes necessary to lower your risk. When you can attach a number, or numbers, to something, it makes it more tangible – and easier to set goals for changing that number.

That's what happened with Anne, the woman quoted at the beginning of this chapter, who found out she had high cholesterol. She immediately started making alterations to her diet to help bring her cholesterol down: substituting non-fat creamer for double cream in her coffee; switching from ordinary ice cream (which she ate almost every night) to low-fat ice cream; and so on. Her cholesterol went from 'too high' to 'desirable'. Specifically, her total cholesterol dropped from 227 to 193 and her LDL-cholesterol went from 141 to 121.

Even women who find that their risk is quite low to start with can use such information to keep doing everything right as far as eating healthily, maintaining a healthy body weight, getting enough exercise and not smoking. It's much easier to keep risk low than to let it creep up and *then* try to decrease it. Likewise, for women who find their risk is moderate or high, it's much easier to bring down the number: the less time time has passed, the less poor habits have become firmly entrenched and the less damage has been done to your arteries.

CHAPTER 4

New Insights: Unravelling the Latest Research

◆

If we could give every individual the right amount of nourishment and exercise, not too little and not too much, we would have found the safest way to health.

— HIPPOCRATES, 460–377 B.C.

This is a great time to be a woman who wants to avoid heart disease. It has been more than twenty years since heart disease began to claim more women's lives each year than men's in the US, yet only in the last decade or so has research into women and cardiovascular health gained enough ground so that specific recommendations for our gender could be formed on the basis of scientific findings. The turning point came in early 1993, when the US government's National Institutes of Health *mandated* that half of all human research be conducted on women.

Before that, the basis for most advice to women about how to lower their heart disease risk had to be extrapolated from findings about men. To be fair, in the 1950s and 1960s, it was men who were losing their lives to heart attacks and related events in the prime of life. And even *they* did not have a huge arsenal of lifestyle strategies at their disposal to reduce the risk of heart disease – or stall it if it had already developed.

For instance, as late as the 1960s, the prevailing thought among many was that vigorous exercise might prove dangerous for people at risk for heart disease. And after someone had a heart attack, the advice was to rest – unlike today, when the advice is most often to get active again as soon as possible. Indeed, the term 'aerobics', which refers to exercises that specifically target the heart and lungs and which everyone now knows, wasn't even coined until the mid-sixties. Until then, the idea of physical activity to protect the heart was limited largely to obscure occupational health studies. In one of them, London bus conductors (all men) who walked up and down the stairs of double-decker buses collecting fares had a lower rate of heart disease deaths than London bus *drivers,* who sat on the job. In another, London postal workers (again, men) with a walking route had a lower level of heart disease than sedentary civil servants – telephonists, executives and clerks, who sat all day.

Some people still feel that research into stemming heart disease isn't as important for women as it is for men because women tend to develop it later in life, after menopause. But that's only partly true. Yes, if a woman develops heart disease, it tends, on average, to be about ten years later than a man. But in the first direct look at the blood vessels of a large group of young women, researchers have discovered that the fatty streaks and artery-clogging plaque that predispose people to heart attacks and other life-threatening coronary events appear in the blood vessels of girls as young as 15.

The investigators who made this finding were involved in a American study called the Pathobiological Determinants in Youth. Their discovery came during autopsies in which they examined the aortas and coronary arteries of young adults who had died from accidents or other untimely causes between the ages of 15 and 34. What they found was that the girls and women had even more extensive amounts of fatty streaks – the beginning of atherosclerotic plaque – than the men. They also found that the presence of *raised* plaque, the type that can start impeding blood flow, increased with age in both women and men. Raised plaque was somewhat more extensive at any given age in men than women, which might help to explain why women exhibit heart disease later in life than men do, but women should not necessarily take comfort in this. Rather, they should take it as motivation to live more heart healthily while still young because it means that they have at least as good a chance as men, if not better, of *slowing* the progression of plaque development.

Research is focused not only on youth but on menopause and beyond as well. As we said in chapter 1, recent findings have shown that hormone replacement therapy (HRT), for decades regarded as protective against heart disease after menopause, is actually linked to a small but significant *increase* in heart disease risk. The US Women's Health Initiative showed that the chances of suffering a heart attack, stroke or life-threatening blood clot increase significantly within months of starting HRT.

That doesn't mean HRT is the wrong choice in the short term for every single woman who is suffering from intolerable hot flushes. But it does mean that, based on the current evidence, it certainly has no benefit in *reducing* the incidence of heart disease and stroke and potentially makes them more likely to occur. It can no longer be viewed as an easy, quick fix.

Also driving the need for a better understanding of how to protect women from heart disease is the fact that it is becoming more common as women, along with the rest of the population, get heavier. As indicated in chapter 3, excess body weight raises your risk for developing heart disease by contributing to increases in LDL-cholesterol levels and blood pressure. It also raises the risk for developing diabetes, which, again, leads to a greater risk for heart disease in women than in men.

What follows is a look at the latest research on the diet and exercise factors that form the basis of the *Strong Women, Strong Hearts* programme. These findings hold great promise and when implemented they can help you take control of your heart health for life.

THE DIETARY UNDERPINNINGS

Scientists have been piecing together those elements of the diet that contribute to heart disease and also those that help to prevent it so that, over time, a clear-cut beneficial eating *pattern* has emerged. There is still much to be learned about how to best tweak the diet to make it more heart-healthy, particularly for women. But we know so much more than we did even ten or twenty years ago.

Literally tens of thousands of investigators worldwide have been participating in the research – the best approach, since an accumulated body of evidence corroborated by many independent investigators is the most reliable. Studies conducted in the Cardiovascular Nutrition Laboratory at Tufts University in the US, directed by Alice Lichtenstein, have made a significant contribution to the scientific findings we have gathered here.

The Fatty Connection

For many years researchers focused on the *amount* of fat in the diet. But now it is clear that the *type* of fat we eat has more to do with our heart disease risk.

Saturated Fat

Even women who have had just a passing interest in nutrition over the years are aware that saturated fat, found in animal foods such as beef, pork and lamb as well as full-fat dairy products like whole milk and cheese, is the biggest dietary contributor to elevated LDL-cholesterol. Researchers started putting together evidence about saturated fat back in the 1950s, although there were hints even before that. Since then the evidence has accumulated, for both women and men. Specifically, when saturated fat is compared head to head in the diet with unsaturated fat, either monounsaturated or polyunsaturated, LDL-cholesterol levels in the blood are higher and the risk of developing heart disease is greater.

Studies in which large numbers of people are observed (frequently referred to as epidemiologic studies) have shown that those individuals who eat the most saturated fat are at the highest risk for developing heart disease. Thus, it's important to keep saturated fat intake low – less than 10 per cent of calories (the limits are actually for saturated fat and *trans*-fatty acids combined, which we'll discuss shortly). If you found your heart disease risk to be at least 10 per cent in chapter 3, then the goal is to keep saturated fat to less than 7 per cent of calories.

You don't need to numerically calculate your percentage of calories from saturated fat. As we'll show you in the next chapter, it's considerably easier than that. You just need to think in terms of foods that contain animal fat versus foods that don't and also *how much* of various foods you eat. That will automatically get you to the right percentages. We'll show you, too, that you can limit saturated fat in your diet and still eat terrific-tasting food.

How much lowering of LDL-cholesterol in your bloodstream can you expect from decreasing the saturated fat in your diet? In one study conducted at Tufts's Cardiovascular Nutrition Laboratory, women who switched from

What's Saturated Fat, Monounsaturated Fat and Polyunsaturated Fat?

Strictly speaking, fats themselves are not saturated, monounsaturated or polyunsaturated. It's certain *components* of fats – fatty acids – that determine their level of saturation. Without dragging anyone back into high school chemistry class, fatty acids are long chains of carbon atoms joined together by either single or double bonds. Saturated fatty acids have no double bonds, monounsaturated have one double bond and polyunsaturated have two or more.

The number of double bonds is critical. Why? In the vast majority of cases, double bonds cause kinks or bends in fatty acids, preventing them from lying flat. In fact, the more double bonds, the more bent the acids are. And that means they can't pile up or pack together like neatly stacked planks of wood. They are more fluid, like uncut logs flowing down a river.

It's for that reason that if a fat has mostly polyunsaturated fatty acids, like soya bean and safflower oil, they won't pack together well and the oil is liquid at room temperature. And if a fat has mostly saturated fatty acids, they will not be bent and therefore will stack up against one another – which is why foods with a lot of saturated fat, like butter, are solid at room temperature. As you will see in chapter 5, saturated fats should be limited as much as possible. Poly- and monounsaturated fats should be used instead.

the typical American diet, which contains about 13 per cent of calories as saturated fat, to a diet with only 7 per cent of calories as saturated fat decreased their LDL-cholesterol by 10 per cent. On average, however, research has shown that decreasing saturated fat intake by 5 per cent of calories and replacing it with the same amount of polyunsaturated fat will reduce LDL-cholesterol levels by about 7 per cent. That's still excellent. Overall, each 1 per cent decrease in cholesterol levels has been associated with a 2 per cent reduction in incidence of coronary heart disease.

Trans-*fatty acids*

A type of fat that is not saturated but which research has shown behaves similarly to saturated fat, or is perhaps slightly more harmful, is *trans* fat. Commonly referred to as *trans*-fatty acids, *trans* fat increases LDL-cholesterol levels. Unlike saturated fat, which also increases HDL-cholesterol levels, *trans* fat does not.

In practical terms, it is a moot point to debate which is worse in our diets because we consume relatively small amounts of *trans* fat compared with saturated fat. However, as with saturated fat, we would still benefit if we decreased intake. Indeed, in a Tufts research project, women who were fed diets that were relatively high in *trans* fat had almost 10 per cent higher LDL-cholesterol levels than women whose diets contained low levels of *trans* fats.

While a small amount of *trans* fat occurs naturally in foods of animal origin, most of it comes from the hydrogenated vegetable oils in processed foods. The process of hydrogenation turns liquid vegetable oils into solids. Think of vegetable shortening and traditional hard margarine.

Now, you may think to yourself, 'I don't cook with shortening or hard margarine, so I don't eat *trans*-fatty acids'. Not true. There are probably still *trans*-fatty acids in your diet. Most of the *trans* fat we eat comes from foods like shop-bought cakes, biscuits, crackers and other items. They also come from fried foods – either from your supermarket's frozen food section or fast-food chains and other restaurants.

Food manufacturers in the UK do not have to label the trans fat in their products, but labels including the words 'hydrogenated vegetable fat' (or oil) or 'partially hydrogenated vegetable fat' will alert you to avoid these items.

This information may be required in the future, however. When you get to the next chapter, you will see that most of the dietary recommendations we make include foods and food ingredients that contain little if any *trans*-fatty acids (and low amounts of saturated fat) to begin with.

Omega-3 Fatty Acids – A Special Kind of Polyunsaturated Fatty Acid

Polyunsaturated fatty acids, in place of saturated and *trans*-fatty acids, definitely help keep blood cholesterol as low as possible. But there are certain types of polyunsaturated fatty acids that outdo others when it comes to protecting the cardiovascular system. Called *omega-3 fatty acids,* they are

Is Olive Oil Better?

With the rise in popularity of the so-called Mediterranean diet, there came a rise in the popularity of olive oil, which is highest not in saturated or polyunsaturated fat but in monounsaturated fat. Fully 77 per cent of the fatty acids in olive oil are monounsaturated, with 14 per cent saturated and 9 per cent polyunsaturated. A lot of people began thinking that if they just added olive oil to their diet, their blood cholesterol problems would be solved.

The same was thought of oils high in polyunsaturated fats in the early 1960s. There are stories of people who went to steak houses and followed up their sirloin entrées with a jigger of corn oil because it was high in polyunsaturated fat, as if one kind of fat could counteract or block the effects of another. It can't. It just adds calories, which leads to weight gain and that generally leads to higher blood cholesterol levels. In other words, adding a particular kind of oil to the diet without subtracting another isn't simply useless – it's harmful.

In short, olive oil itself doesn't *lower* cholesterol levels, as some people believe. It lowers them only if you use it *in place of* saturated fat. And, as it turns out, research has shown that *other* vegetable oils, such as rapeseed, which is lower in saturated fat than olive oil, is even more effective. So are soya bean oil and corn oil, which are particularly high in polyunsaturated fat.

None of this is to say you shouldn't use olive oil. You should use it if you like the flavour. The two of us keep several types of oil in our houses: olive oil for salads, safflower or rapeseed oil for cooking and a little sesame oil for flavouring dishes with an Asian twist.

contained in fish and go under the names EPA (eicosapentaenoic acid) and DHA (docosahexaenoic acid).

EPA and DHA don't generally affect LDL-cholesterol levels. They appear to work in other ways. For instance, in one study recently published in the *American Journal of Clinical Nutrition* (called the Estrogen, Regression and

Atherosclerosis study, or ERA), it was demonstrated that women with diabetes who had already had a heart attack experienced a slower rate of atherosclerosis progression than similar women if they ate at least two fish meals a week or one fish meal that contained cold-water fish such as salmon or tuna. This was the first study in women to show a direct relationship between fish and slowed progression of atherosclerotic disease.

Other evidence in women indicates that those who eat *any* healthily prepared fish, even as infrequently as a couple of times a month, have reduced rates of heart disease. Furthermore, if they suffer a coronary event, they are less likely to die.

Still other research suggests that the fat in fish makes blood platelets less 'sticky' and therefore less likely to aggregate and form clots. It also appears to decrease the propensity of the heart to beat abnormally, a condition known as arrhythmia. Finally, fish promotes the relaxation of the lining of the blood vessels, which allows blood to flow more freely. In some people, it mildly decreases blood pressure.

Fatty, cold-water fish such as salmon seem to be more protective than white-flesh fish like cod. One reason, of course, is that fatty fish have more omega-3s. But also, white-fleshed fish is frequently battered and fried, which adds saturated (or sometimes *trans*) fat – and calories – that work to cancel out the effect of any omega-3s present. We will discuss some delicious ways to prepare fish healthily in the next chapter.

Fish is not the only source of omega-3 fatty acids. They are also found in rapeseed, soya bean and walnut oil, as well as in walnuts. But the body has to convert the omega-3s in those foods to the heart-healthy EPA and DHA contained in fish. And it converts them inefficiently, at a rate of 10 per cent or less. Still, these oils and nuts are reasonable choices as part of a heart-healthy dietary pattern. Milk supplemented with omega-3 is also available now.

How Low Should Fat Go?
You may have heard that fat should make up no more than 30 per cent of calories. But in the last couple of years, that guideline has been liberalized. It's okay for fat to comprise up to 35 per cent of calories – as long as saturated fat and *trans*-fatty acids *combined* don't make up more than 10 per cent of calories. We're not necessarily *advocating* a diet that gets 35 per cent of calories from fat. A gram of fat contains more than twice as many calories as a

gram of carbohydrate or protein, so it can be easy to go overboard on calories on a somewhat high-fat diet. It's simply that if calories on a higher-fat diet can be kept low enough to keep you at a healthy weight and it is the right kind of fat – polyunsaturated and monounsaturated and fat from fish – going up to 35 per cent of calories as fat is not harmful.

At least as important, you should not go on a very low-fat diet, one in which less than 20 per cent of calories come from fat. As fat intake goes down, carbohydrate intake goes up and it has been well established that a very high-carbohydrate diet can raise triglyceride levels and keep down HDL-cholesterol. Consider that in one research trial, women and men whose diets were 29 per cent fat had normal trigylceride levels averaging 115 and HDL-cholesterol concentrations averaging 42. But when fat was reduced to 15 per cent of calories, triglycerides shot up to an average of 188 and HDL-cholesterol dropped to an average of 35.

The bottom line is: stick to a diet both moderate in fat and unprocessed carbohydrates – fruits, vegetables, legumes and whole grains.

Counting Cholesterol

There has been a lot of confusion over cholesterol in the diet. Many people assume that the cholesterol in the foods you eat – eggs, meat and full-fat dairy products like whole milk, butter and ice cream – contributes directly to the amount of cholesterol in your bloodstream. Not true. Scientists have known for decades that how cholesterol gets into your blood is quite complex. In fact, saturated fat and *trans*-fatty acids are the major dietary determinants of cholesterol in your bloodstream, not the cholesterol you eat.

That said, the cholesterol in foods *can* increase blood cholesterol to some degree, more in some people than in others depending on genetics. Thus, if you're told you have elevated LDL-cholesterol, you should keep your dietary cholesterol at a maximum of 200 milligrams a day. Fortunately, if you're already following a diet that's low in saturated fat, that's easy to do. Most cholesterol-containing foods are also foods that contain a fair amount of saturated fat. (Eggs, which we'll discuss in the next chapter, are an exception.)

The Carbohydrate Connection

Forget everything you've heard about carbohydrates making you fat. They don't – unless you eat too many of them. But that's true of anything.

What's important to keep in mind about carbohydrates when it comes to heart disease is that certain carbohydrate-rich foods have clearly been associated with a decreased risk. The foods we're talking about are vegetables, fruits and wholegrain items like wholegrain breads and cereals.

Why is not completely clear. As we said in chapter 3, it may have something to do with the fact that these foods all contain fibre, which is associated with better weight management and therefore with a reduced risk for heart problems. Fibre takes up a fair amount of room in the gut and apparently has the ability to help people feel sated even though it doesn't contain any calories.

Research has also shown that fibre helps keep down blood glucose and, to a small extent, helps lower blood cholesterol. In the ERA study, women who had suffered a heart attack and subsequently ate at least 3 grams of fibre from wholegrain foods every day, such as cereals and wholewheat bread, experienced slower progression of atherosclerotic plaque afterwards than women who consumed less fibre.

Some studies have even suggested that fibre decreases blood pressure. But it's also important to note that people who eat plenty of high-fibre foods have less room in their diets for high-calorie foods that can contribute to increased weight – and increased blood pressure.

Whatever the mechanism by which fibre works, hundreds, if not thousands, of studies have consistently shown a link between diets high in produce and low rates of chronic disease, including cardiovascular disease. It's the same for diets high in whole grains and produce.

The Protein Connection: Soya Story

While the kinds and amounts of carbohydrates and fats people eat can vary widely and have a significant effect on heart disease risk, Americans consume a pretty constant level of protein: about 15 per cent of total calories (unless they follow one of the high-protein diets, which we don't recommend). While the type of fat the protein comes packaged with is important (there is saturated fat in beef, for instance, and largely unsaturated fat in fish), the protein itself doesn't have as much to do with heart health as is often thought – or written about in the press.

For a while it was believed that protein from soya-based foods such as tofu could significantly lower the chance of developing heart disease by lowering blood cholesterol, even to the point that in the US claims for reduced heart-disease risk are now allowed on soya-containing foods. But while soya foods do make excellent protein substitutes for animal foods because they have virtually no saturated fat, the evidence that soya protein itself lowers cholesterol is much weaker than was originally thought. In one study conducted by Alice's group at the Cardiovascular Nutrition Laboratory, women and men who were fed a minimum of 50 grams of soya protein a day reduced their LDL-cholesterol by just 2 per cent compared to those who were fed foods like steak and chicken instead. And 50 grams is a *lot* – the equivalent of almost 700 grams of tofu.

A similar but larger study conducted in Scandinavia recently corroborated this finding – and has also found that soya protein does not protect bone density (or cognitive function).

Specific Vitamins and Minerals

Fat, carbohydrates and protein are known as the three macronutrients. They are the only nutrients that contribute calories to our diets (along with alcohol). There are also the micronutrients – vitamins and minerals – and emerging research has turned up some intriguing information on whether some of them can help stave off heart disease. In some cases, the findings have been promising. In others, the evidence of benefit has not been as strong as researchers originally hoped. In still other cases, the jury remains out. Whatever the evidence, it's important always to bear in mind that it's the dietary *pattern* that counts, not any particular nutrient in isolation. But it's good to know which single nutrients might be having an effect because it allows that pattern to be tailored to the best possible advantage.

B Vitamins

People who follow diets high in the B vitamins folate, B_6 and B_{12} have relatively low levels in the blood of homocysteine, a substance implicated in heart disease risk that we discussed in chapter 2. While the research is ongoing and we don't yet know whether reducing homocysteine levels by eating more foods with B vitamins actually reduces heart disease risk (we have got from point X to point Y but not from point Y to point Z), these vitamins are found in foods that belong in a heart-healthy eating pattern anyway. Folate, for instance, is contained in legumes such as kidney beans, chickpeas and lentils, along with green leafy vegetables and orange juice. In the UK it is also found in bread made with fortified flour, and fortified breakfast cereals, but these can also contain a high sugar content. Vitamin B_6 is plentiful in vegetables as well as in fruits and can also be found in seafood, poultry and beef. And B_{12} is in all foods of animal origin. Thus, if you're eating right, B vitamins are keeping down homocysteine automatically, which is a 'can't-hurt, might-help' part of the bargain.

Vitamin K

Found in highest concentrations in green leafy vegetables, vitamin K is now thought possibly to contribute to heart health in ways previously unidentified. Researchers in the Vitamin K Laboratory at Tufts University are currently investigating whether it can help slow hardening of the arteries. There's already test tube and animal research that suggests as much. To test it in humans, investigators are giving more than 450 people either 500 micrograms of vitamin K every day or a placebo, or dummy pill. They will then look at their degree of vascular calcification later on down the line.

Currently, Americans consume an average of about 120 micrograms of vitamin K daily. But it's easy to get more. A half cup of cooked spinach contains 360 micrograms; a half cup of Brussels sprouts (which amounts to just four sprouts), 235 micrograms; and a half cup of cooked collard greens, 400 micrograms. Even if vitamin K doesn't ultimately prove to protect against heart disease, eating more of these green vegetables is consistent with eating heart-healthily in general.

Calcium

When it comes to heart disease, calcium falls into the same category as vitamin K. The research suggests but doesn't prove that this nutrient may have something to do with reduced risk. Specifically, there's a body of research that suggests calcium might help regulate blood pressure, especially when consumed as part of a diet high in fruits and vegetables. Some research, albeit extremely thin, even suggests it may be associated with helping to keep down blood cholesterol.

The good news here: you don't need to wait for definitive results before you incorporate more calcium in your diet. *All* women should eat at least two, preferably three, servings of high-calcium foods every day anyway, to avoid osteoporosis. Skimmed and 1 per cent milk, low- and non-fat yo-gurt, canned salmon or sardines with the bones, many brands of tofu and soya milk (check the nutrition labels), 25 to 40 grams of hard cheese, cal-cium-fortified juices and cereals – all of these fill the bill as high-calcium choices. Smaller but still significant amounts of calcium can be found in broccoli, oranges, figs and other plant-based foods.

Vitamin E

Hopes were originally very high for the role of vitamin E supplements in preventing heart disease, so much so that many doctors still recommend it to their patients. But while observations of large populations suggested a pro-tective effect from vitamin E supplements, numerous carefully controlled studies in which some people were given vitamin E pills and others a placebo have not panned out. The E takers were no more protected from future heart attacks and other cardiovascular events than the non–E takers. (As far as vitamin E and immune function along with protection against cancer, the jury is still out, despite claims in ads and the popular press.)

Potassium

The US National Academy of Sciences recommends that people consume 4,700 milligrams of potassium daily. That's the amount deemed necessary for helping to stave off high blood pressure. Potassium is found mostly in fruits and vegetables (see page 67). Currently, Americans, including women, average only about 2,300 milligrams of potassium a day.

To raise it high enough, it would be necessary to double produce con-sumption from the current national average of four to five servings a day to eight to ten servings daily.

That's exactly what the DASH diet suggests. DASH is an acronym for Di-etary Approaches to Stop Hypertension, an eating plan that so successfully lowered blood pressure in research studies that it has been endorsed by the National Heart, Lung and Blood Institute in the US.

The Details Come Together in the DASH Diet

In 1997 scientists from six major medical centres around the US first tested the DASH diet. In that trial, participants were provided with a diet containing eight to ten daily servings of fruits and vegetables, two to three servings of low-fat dairy foods and a couple of small portions of meat, chicken or fish – all of which ensured that they were consuming plenty of potassium, calcium, B vitamins and other nutrients that research has found look promising for preventing heart disease in general. The upshot: the DASH diet was significantly more effective at lowering blood pressure than the typical American diet that is low in produce as well as high-calcium dairy items. In a follow-up study in 2000, the researchers went a step further, putting people on essentially the same DASH diet but manipulating certain foods so that the study participants were at one of three sodium levels: 3,300 milligrams a day (about as much as many women eat); 2,400 milligrams a day (less than many women consume); or 1,500 milligrams a day (less than virtually anyone in the US eats). It turned out that the lower the sodium level, the more blood pressure dropped – even for people whose blood pressure started out in the normal or high-normal ranges. That's important because generally speaking, the lower your blood pressure, the lower your risk for stroke and heart disease.

With some tweaking to reflect findings about heart disease prevention that have come out since the DASH diet was tested, the recommendations of our dietary plan in the next chapter largely coincide with the recommendations of DASH: plenty of produce and low-fat dairy products, modest portions of meat and little in the way of sweets and salty snacks. And because our plan is based largely on whole foods that have not gone through a lot of processing, it's naturally low in sodium.

THE EXERCISE UNDERPINNINGS

Diet is *half* of what you need to focus on, lifestyle-wise, to protect your heart. The other half is physical activity. Researchers are coming to understand, in fact, that the two together are absolutely vital for the best heart health possible. Yes, you have to eat correctly to treat your arteries and heart well. But if you don't challenge your body by working it through exercise, your heart muscle and the rest of your cardiovascular system will not work at their best levels. All the good eating in the world, while crucial in its own right, isn't enough to counteract a sedentary lifestyle.

Aerobics

In 1968, Dr Kenneth Cooper published a book called *Aerobics,* both coining a new term and marking the beginning of a fitness revolution. Aerobics – brisk walking, running, swimming, biking and other activities during which the body is in continuous motion – challenges your heart, lungs and entire vascular system to work harder and thereby makes them stronger and more efficient at their jobs. People who participate regularly in aerobics have lower heart rates, which, as you'll recall from chapter 2, means they need fewer beats per minute to pump oxygen- and nutrient-rich blood from the heart to the rest of the body.

But it wasn't until ten years after Dr Cooper's book came out – 1978 – that aerobics was put on the scientific map as a significant contributor to reduced risk of heart disease. That year, a researcher from Stanford University named Ralph Paffenbarger, MD, published a remarkable study in the *Journal of Epidemiology.* He and his colleagues had studied almost 17,000 Harvard alumni (all men) ages 35 to 74. All had entered Harvard sometime between 1916 and 1950.

Using answers to questionnaires, Dr Paffenbarger and his colleagues learned that more than 500 of the men had already had a heart attack. They also learned how many stairs the men climbed and how far they walked daily as well as to what degree they participated in strenuous sports. In other words, they got an insight on the men's current degree of aerobic activity. What the researchers found was that the men who burned at least 2,000 calories a week in aerobic activities were 64 per cent less likely to have been one of the heart attack sufferers. They also found – and this is crucial – that the men's current aerobic habits were much more predictive of their heart health than their physical activity patterns while they were in college. Having been athletic decades before doesn't offset a sedentary lifestyle now. Or, put more positively, becoming aerobically active in middle or old age has a lot more bearing on your heart health than having been sedentary in your twenties. Age matters less; it's what you do today that counts.

But Do the Findings Apply Directly to Women?

At around the same time that US west-coast researchers at Stanford were finding that exercise protects men's hearts, east-coast investigators at Harvard were gearing up to start the long-running Nurses' Health Study, which began in the late 1970s with almost 122,000 female nurses from around the country who were between 30 and 55. The study was originally set up to look at the health effects of the birth control pill. But the scientists quickly realized they were working with an enormously rich resource for studying issues in women that hadn't yet been systematically studied – diet, exercise, body weight and smoking, and the effect of those lifestyle factors on disease, health and longevity. Here are some of the findings, reported intermittently over the years, as the study went (and continues to go) forwards:

- Women who walk at a brisk pace for at least three hours a week reduce their risk for heart attacks and other coronary events by 35 per cent compared to women who walk only infrequently. The same holds true for reducing their risk for diabetes.
- Women who engage in the most physical activity each week – equivalent to about a half hour a day of very brisk walking – are at a 34 per cent decreased risk of suffering a stroke compared to those who exercise the least.
- Physical activity helps to protect women from heart disease even if they are at high risk because they are overweight or they smoke. They are not as well protected as exercisers who are of normal weight and don't smoke, but they are significantly more protected than sedentary overweight women and smokers.

The Nurses' Health Study isn't the only one that links women's cardiovascular health to physical activity. The Cooper Institute for Aerobics Research in Dallas now has data on more than 40,000 women and men combined. The first and most classic research paper on some of them appeared in 1989 in the *Journal of the American Medical Association.* In an eight-year study that included more than 3,000 women and 10,000 men, it was found that those in the bottom 20 per cent of fitness ranking were 65 per cent more likely to die from heart attacks and strokes (and diabetes and cancer!) than the 20 per cent of people in the top fitness ranking, as measured by treadmill test performance.

Johns Hopkins Medical Institutions researcher Samia Mora, MD, obtained corroborating findings in her research just a couple of years ago. Almost 3,000 women aged 30 to 80 with no symptoms indicative of a bad heart underwent treadmill tests in the 1970s. They were observed for exercise capacity – how intensely they could go at it on a treadmill – and also for the amount of time it took for their heartbeats to return to normal after they stopped exercising. Twenty years later, those who had not been able to work up to an intensity equivalent to walking about five miles an hour (which is a very brisk pace) and whose heart rates did not 'recover' by declining towards resting rate by at least 55 beats per minute were three and a half times more likely than those with better numbers to have died of heart disease – or *any* other cause. **Exercise ability was so strongly linked with the risk of death that even a sedentary woman who had desirable blood cholesterol levels, didn't smoke and didn't have high blood pressure was at six times the risk of dying from heart disease as a very active woman with the same desirable cholesterol and blood pressure.**

The upside here is: exercise capacity, or fitness, can be improved significantly even with moderate physical activity in just a matter of months. It goes back to the fact that even if you've been inactive your whole life, you can dramatically lower your risk of dying prematurely simply by walking briskly or engaging in other aerobic activities on a regular basis *now*. You'll lower your blood pressure (as dozens of clinical trials have shown) and blood cholesterol (as dozens of other trials have shown), not to mention help control your weight, improve your overall function and quality of life and get better-quality sleep.

No wonder the US Surgeon General, the Dietary Guidelines for Americans and the American Heart Association all say that people should set a goal of at least 30 minutes of moderate-intensity physical activity (15 to 20 minutes per mile) on most (preferably all) days of the week. Even more cardiovascular gains will be accrued by exercising *vigorously* for 20 to 40 minutes three to five days per week – to the point where you break a sweat.

Unfortunately, as awareness about the benefits of aerobic activity has increased, actual participation in aerobics has levelled off after increasing through the sixties, seventies and eighties. Only 27 per cent of Americans get enough exercise to benefit them and 38 per cent of American women are not active at all.

Aerobic Exercise Starts Working *Immediately*

Of course, the more frequently you exercise, the greater the bene-fits to your heart. But some effects are immediate. Consider that triglycerides are reduced right away by vigorous exercise and that the effects last up to seventy-two hours. Similarly, exercise causes transient increases in HDL-cholesterol, reduces blood pressure for up to twelve hours and improves glucose uptake by the cells.

And preliminary evidence suggests that just a single bout of exercise helps your heart rate become more variable. Why would you want your heart rate to become more variable?

The reason, new research suggests, is that women who have a very stable, nonvarying resting heart rate (*beat, beat, beat*) are at greater risk for cardiac events – and death – than women whose resting heart rate keeps shifting (*beat, beat, beatbeat, beat*). A steady, unchanging heart rate means your heart is not able to respond to tiny fluctuations in body processes. A heart that can adapt to and accommodate the body's subtle changes in needs moment to moment can help keep things more finely tuned.

Sedentary women who are older are particularly apt to have com-promised heart rate variability; over time, there is a decline in the ability of the heart to react moment by moment to changes in the need for blood flow and oxygen in the rest of the body. But, and this is a big but, when a team of scientists in France set out to evaluate the impact that exercise has on heart rate variability in adults with an average age of 75, they found that those who were regularly active had signifi-cantly higher heart rate variability than their more unfit counter-parts. The bottom line: with exercise you can become young at heart, literally, improving the heart muscle's ability to adapt quickly and thereby help reduce the risk of a heart attack, stroke or other cardio-vascular calamity.

Strength Training

When you think about exercising for heart health, the chances are that you think about aerobic activities like walking and bicycling, which makes sense, since they directly affect heart and lung capacity. But more and more research is bringing to light the fact that strength training improves heart health, too.

The most obvious reason is that strength training improves aerobic capabilities. Former Tufts colleagues of ours proved this point when they studied patients in a local cardiac rehabilitation programme. All the patients participated in walking several times weekly, but only half of them did strength training three times a week. After twenty-one weeks, the aerobic gains made by the strength trainers were 18 per cent greater. Why? When you increase the strength of your muscles, including your leg muscles, through strength training, walking becomes easier. That, in turn, lets you walk faster and farther, which gives the heart and lungs a better workout.

But strength training does more than allow for better aerobic training. Studies have also shown that people who lift weights regularly have lower blood pressure. One study was conducted here at Tufts by Carmen Castaneda, MD, a close colleague of Miriam's. After sixteen weeks, women and men who had been enrolled in a strength-training programme experienced significant reductions in blood pressure. They also lost fat around the abdomen, which presents more of a heart disease risk than fat on the hips, thighs and buttocks.

Perhaps most important, the participants, all of whom had diabetes, experienced significant improvements in blood sugar – to the point that most of them were able to reduce their diabetes medication. That's no small achievement since, as we've noted, diabetes itself greatly increases the risk for heart disease.

It has been common knowledge for many years that exercise helps control diabetes. But the research has generally looked at aerobic exercise. Now we know that strength training is a critical element in the arsenal of lifestyle approaches to help women control this disease. (The information comes none too soon. In the United States diabetes is on the rise, with a 700 per cent increase since 1960. An estimated 16 million Americans have it and another

17 million are pre-diabetic. And the age at which people are getting it, because of increasing weight coupled with increasing physical inactivity, is getting younger and younger. It's no longer just a condition of middle and old age.)

As for strength training's ability to reduce the rate of heart disease directly, results from trials on women are still pending. But in a Harvard study of more than 40,000 men, it was found that those who did strength training more than thirty minutes a week had a reduction in cardiovascular risk of about 30 per cent. We suspect the same will be found true in women.

Strength training does not take as much time as aerobics. Twice a week, thirty to forty minutes per session, will suffice.

DIET AND EXERCISE: THE WHOLE PACKAGE

The best part about the heart-healthy benefits of the right dietary patterns and the right kinds of exercise is that they are all in your hands. That is, research has proven unequivocally that whether or not you substantially decrease your risk for heart disease is very much up to you. You're not 'stuck' with a particular heart disease risk because of your genes or your family history or because 'things are the way they are'. Indeed, the scientific evidence from the 100,000-plus women in the US Nurses' Health Study suggests that women who eat a healthy diet and exercise regularly (and don't smoke and maintain a desirable body weight) can enjoy up to an 84 per cent reduction in the risk of cardiovascular death.

Yet only 3 per cent of the women studied were in that heart-healthy lifestyle category. In fact, as we alluded to earlier, the American lifestyle has become so far removed from what is good for us that deaths from poor diet and inactivity will soon overtake deaths from smoking.

We hope to change those numbers dramatically. In the next section, we give clear, detailed instructions for how to translate the dietary and exercise research into a lifestyle you can live with – and enjoy! You'll see that eating well and incorporating more physical activity into your days will feel so good, you'll never want to return to your old habits.

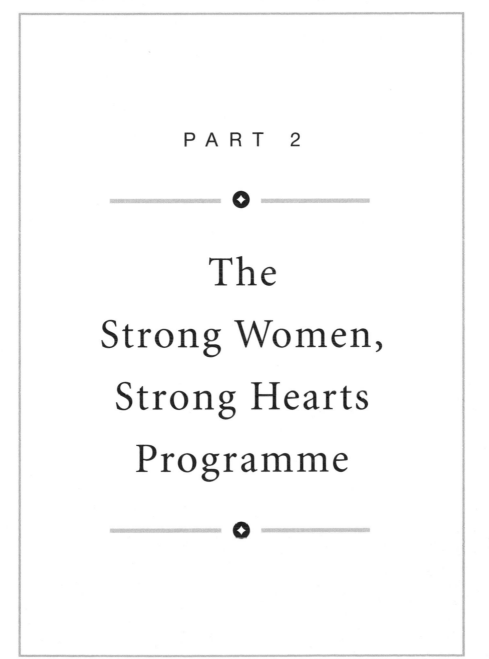

PART 2

The
Strong Women,
Strong Hearts
Programme

CHAPTER 5

Don't Think Diet –
Think Food Patterns

◆

I had let everything go. Before menopause, my cholesterol used to be really low. After, it was much higher. At the same time, I was eating all the bad stuff – too many desserts, too much sugar, too many biscuits. I needed to get back on the bandwagon and start eating real food. I started by eating more fruits and vegetables, drinking mostly water if I was thirsty. Now I eat a lot of salads. I put in currants or pine nuts or sunflower seeds, avocado, tomato, spring onions, cucumber. Maybe a little bit of crumbled feta cheese. And I dress it with olive oil, a little balsamic vinegar, garlic and a splash of lemon juice. I realized I wasn't going to stick with it if it was too boring. I didn't want to eat just plain vegetables. I wanted it to be interesting. It had to taste good and I had to be able to look forward to it.

– WENDY

Conjure up the word 'diet' and the words 'restrictive', 'punishing', 'boring' and 'lacking flavour' won't be far behind. That's because so often, when health professionals as well as the media talk about diet, they talk about things you shouldn't eat, foods you can no longer enjoy. It's as though the whole world has become the proverbial finger-wagging lady with a hair net in the school cafeteria, the one who has nothing tasty to offer and heaps limp, overcooked green beans onto your plate with a scowl.

The 'food-can't-taste-good' notion is especially deep-rooted when it comes to diets for preventing disease. After all, if you want to keep your heart healthy into old age and also substantially stunt unhealthy rises in blood pressure, there has to be an onerous trade-off, right? Stay away from fat, stay away from meat, watch this, watch that.

Well, guess what? Eating for heart health happens to be delicious, as we both know firsthand and will show you with menu ideas and recipe suggestions. Heart-healthy eating is taste, it's texture, it's colour – it's enjoyment. As well it must be. As Wendy says, if you don't like what you eat, your eating plan will backfire because it will not become your default mode – what you automatically do instead of what you *have* to do. Sure, you may experience an episodic burst of enthusiasm for a diet you don't like because you feel motivated, initially, to take care of your health. But if you have to give up too much in the way of gustatory satisfaction or it becomes too cumbersome to adhere to in your everyday life, that enthusiasm is going to wane – fast – and you'll be back where you started.

More good news about a heart-healthy diet: on top of its being something you'll be *glad* to incorporate into your lifestyle, following it will protect not just your heart health but also your health in general. That's right. Eating heart healthily will decrease your risk of developing diabetes, hypertension, some cancers, osteoporosis and a host of other ills – for *anyone*. If you're raising children or sharing your life with a significant other, you will be imprinting important health-promoting behaviour onto the lifestyle template of those you love.

YOU DON'T NEED A DEGREE IN SCIENCE TO DO THIS

In the previous chapter, we went through a good deal of research to show you the bases of our recommendations. But you don't need to be a scientific investigator to eat right, constantly counting milligrams or calculating percentages. Putting our nutrition programme into practice is deceptively *un*complicated. It will work no matter what your eating style – meat eater, vegetarian or somewhere in between. That's because it is really a dietary *pattern* rather than prescriptions for or against particular foods and so can be adapted to accommodate almost any dietary preferences or restrictions. It simply involves keeping the emphasis on the whole foods available on the perimeter of the

Is There Such a Thing as a Cholesterol-Lowering Food?

Are there really foods that can legitimately be called *cholesterol lowerers*? For instance, one often hears that oatmeal is a cholesterol-lowering food.

We don't believe it's a good idea to think of individual foods that way. Foods don't work in isolation. They work in concert with all the other foods you eat. That is, you can't eat a bowl of oatmeal and follow it up with a hot fudge sundae and expect to lower your blood cholesterol. A food can only work as well as the whole nutrition plan it's fit into.

Thus, when you read or hear that a single food is good for the heart, the questions you have to ask yourself are: what am I going to give up if I add in the new food? Is it high in saturated fat or *trans-fatty acids*? Low in fibre? Will I be forgoing as many calories as I'm going to be consuming with the new item? If you decide the food is a good choice for you, then by all means include it in your heart-healthy eating plan – if you happen to like it.

Keep in mind that if you're already eating a healthy pattern of foods that don't contain too many calories and have plenty of fibre and other healthy components, making room for one particular food isn't going to make all that much difference. And if you're not eating well to begin with, adding that food won't overcome the overall shortcomings, either. It takes more than one food to change your food-eating pattern.

supermarket (the produce and dairy aisles, for instance) rather than on the boxed, bagged, canned and other packaged goods lining all the centre aisles. Those choices often contain too little fibre, too many refined carbohydrates that lack certain nutrients and frequently too much in the way of sugar, saturated and *trans* fats and salt. Stick to whole and minimally processed foods and, sooner than you think, they will become the choices you *want*, not the way you have to eat.

Wendy puts it this way: 'I got to a point where I wanted to eat as "real" as I could, instead of eating quick, fast junk. I soon found I wasn't eating things from bottles, jars and packets. I literally had less rubbish to put out. The good stuff isn't just going to appear in your refrigerator. You have to watch what you put there; you have to make the shift. But once you start to do it, it's just like junk food – it becomes a habit.'

That doesn't mean you can never have some potato crisps or packaged convenience food ever again. *Any* food can fit into a heart-healthy diet, at least once in a while. It just means that most of your choices will have undergone little to no tampering at a food-processing plant.

To keep the focus on the delicious, nutrient-dense foods that will form the centrepiece of your heart-healthy eating plan, keep in mind this HEART acronym:

H eap on the vegetables and fruits.
E mphasize the right fats.
A ccentuate whole grains.
R evere low- and non-fat dairy foods.
T arget heart-healthy proteins.

Now we'll take a closer look at each of these points.

Heap on the Vegetables and Fruits

GOAL: seven to nine servings daily

SERVING SIZE: 1 cup raw leafy vegetables, such as lettuce or spinach
1 cup raw vegetables, cut up
½ cup cooked vegetables
¾ cup vegetable juice
1 medium fruit, such as an apple, pear or orange
1 cup raw fruit (sliced or chopped)
1 cup berries, grapes or other small fruit
½ cup cooked, frozen or canned (in its own juice) fruit
¼ cup dried fruit
¾ cup 100% fruit juice

Vegetable and Fruit Powerhouses

Fibre-Rich

All vegetables and fruits (but not juices) are good sources of fibre. Below are some particularly high-fibre choices. The Recommended Daily Allowance for fibre is 25 grams. (Remember, some of your fibre will also come from whole grains and beans.)

	Grams of fibre
1 cup raspberries	8
1 pear	4
1 cup blueberries	4
1 apple	4
½ cup cooked peas	4
½ cup cooked Brussels sprouts	3
1 orange	3
½ cup cooked spinach	3
1 banana	3
1 small baked potato with skin	3

Plenty of Potassium

The recommendation for potassium is 4,700 milligrams. (Currently, Americans average about 2,500 milligrams.) Following are some particularly potassium-rich vegetables and fruits. (Other nutritious foods are good sources of potassium, too. A cup of plain yogurt has 531 milligrams; 85g of cooked halibut or tuna steak, almost 500 milligrams.)

	Milligrams of potassium
1 small baked potato with skin	593
1 cup cantaloupe chunks	494
1 baked sweet potato with skin	493
1 banana	467
½ cup cooked winter squash	448
½ cup cooked spinach	420
¾ cup orange juice	355

If we were designing our own food guide pyramid, vegetables and fruits, rather than grains, would form the base. What makes us feel so strongly here is the *consistency* with which studies have shown that diets rich in vegetables and fruits are associated with a decreased risk for developing heart disease and stroke.

How many servings of produce should you be eating a day? The standard advice is at least five, but we believe there is good reason to eat more in the order of seven to nine. At the very least, that much will get you closer to the 25 grams of fibre that adults should eat daily. And produce is low in calories compared to many other types of foods. Therefore, if it becomes a mainstay in your diet, you will have a better shot at successful weight management by virtue of its replacing other, higher-calorie options. Produce is also high in potassium and generally very low in sodium, both of which are associated with decreased blood pressure.

Note that we say 'vegetables and fruits', not 'fruits and vegetables'. This is not by chance. Fruits are great for you, but vegetables, in particular, tend to be nutrient-rich and are hard to overdo because they're relatively low in calories. We recommend at least four to five servings of vegetables daily and two to four of fruit, preferably not in the form of juice.

If you really love 175ml of orange or grapefruit juice in the morning and you don't have a weight problem, fine. But whole fruit, unlike juice, offers fibre. And it tends to be more filling. An orange will stave off mid-morning hunger much better than a glass of orange juice. (We'll explain further in chapter 7.)

Incorporating more produce into your diet is not hard *at all*, especially when you consider that frozen is just as nutritious as fresh and is easy to keep in the house. As you buy it in bags you can always take from the freezer as much or as little as you like. Tips for increasing vegetables and fruits throughout the day:

- Heat some frozen spinach, broccoli or sliced Brussels sprouts in the microwave or on the stove to have with dinner or to top a toasted wholewheat sourdough roll with melted cheese for lunch.
- Make a chicken salad that's half chopped celery and shredded carrots and half chicken.
- Into either your own homemade tomato sauce or into prepared sauce, toss finely chopped or grated vegetables. This is great for

Potatoes: A Vegetable or a Starch?

Potatoes have been much maligned in recent years as bad 'carbs' that will send your blood sugar soaring and make you fat. Don't be too quick to judge. Potatoes are decent vegetables that have been unfairly criticized. Their skin is a good source of fibre and the fleshy part contains lots of potassium and a reasonable amount of vitamin C, along with other nutrients.

Potatoes *are* starchier than other vegetables, meaning they do have a lot of carbohydrates, similar to grains. In fact, culturally and culinarily, they are generally used as a starch rather than as a vegetable per se. And like starches, they also contain more calories than other vegetables gram for gram. For example, there are 26 calories in 25 grams of baked potato, compared with only 7 in 25 grams of cooked broccoli. That totals 128 calories for a smallish potato and much more if potatoes are turned into French fries – the way a lot of potatoes are consumed in Britain and the US. Along with calories, fries usually contain *trans*-fatty acids because of the fat they are fried in.

Even if you eat a potato baked rather than fried, adding a lot of butter and sour cream cuts into its healthiness by making it much more calorific – and not the best choice for your heart because those toppings are extremely high in saturated fat.

For that reason, we suggest that you use small baked potatoes (preferably with the skin), or split a larger one between two people, topping it with a little low-fat sour cream, or perhaps low-fat yogurt mixed with chives. And think of potatoes as a grain rather than a vegetable. That is, they're not 'instead of' broccoli; they're instead of bread, rice or pasta.

Keep in mind, too, that potatoes are only one tasty side-dish starch. There are lots of wholegrain starches that are delicious but that people make too little use of, as you'll see on page 72, in 'Accentuate Whole Grains'.

family members who aren't big on produce because it doesn't change the taste much.

- Consider adding vegetables where they may not have been before. For example, if preparing lasagna, mix thawed chopped spinach with the ricotta cheese. Or slice an aubergine into 0.5cm slices, drizzle on vegetable oil, bake at 200°C until soft and use as its own lasagna layer.
- Keep frozen berries on hand to top yogurt or ice cream. Just thaw them in the microwave before using.
- Toss a handful of dried cranberries into a green salad with feta cheese and vinaigrette.
- Make one of Miriam's one-minute fruit smoothies for an afternoon snack: throw into the blender 225ml of non-fat yogurt, 75g of frozen berries or other frozen fruit of your choice and a splash of blueberry or grape juice; blend for 30 seconds and hey presto!

We are fortunate that more and more fruits are available at reasonable prices year-round. Always keep a bowl of fruit within easy reach. For fruit that ripens quickly, such as peaches and nectarines, put out only a few at a time. Better to have a small bowl with a limited number of fruits that look good in order to make them more appealing. If you do this, fruit will become the default snack.

It's that way with produce in general. Availability translates into consumption. If you always have fresh, frozen or canned on hand, you'll eat it (and may even eat less of other foods that aren't so heart-healthy).

Emphasize the Right Fats

Given the typical western diet, the first order of the day is to reduce consumption of heart-unhealthy fats. That includes the saturated fat in beef, poultry and other meat as well as full-fat dairy foods and the *trans*-fatty acids in commercially fried and baked foods and other items, including the legions of packaged foods that run the gamut from biscuits, cakes and crackers to microwavable popcorn and frozen entrées.

But you can also improve your diet by choosing the fats, or oils, most conducive to heart health. As we said before, a low-fat diet is no longer considered the right way to go. It's a *moderate*-fat diet, as long as you have the right fats.

The omega-3 fatty acids in fish are a great help, of course.

When it comes to cooking, the best bets are most vegetable oils. These include rapeseed, safflower, sunflower, corn, olive and soya bean oil. Rapeseed is the lowest in saturated fat of all cooking oils, with all the others close behind. When we say 'vegetable oil', we are always referring to one of these, any of which is heart-healthy. We think it's best to keep a few different types in the house for particular uses, such as sautéeing vegetables, dressing salads and so on.

Nutrition researchers as well as public health experts used to make a big distinction between oils high in monounsaturated fatty acids, such as olive

Are Nuts Especially Heart Healthy?

You may have heard a lot about nuts recently. There's even a health claim about them, approved by the US Food and Drug Administration, saying they might help reduce the risk for heart disease: 'Scientific evidence suggests but does not prove that eating 40 grams per day of most nuts as part of a diet low in saturated fat and cholesterol may reduce the risk of heart disease'. It's true that nuts, like other plant-based foods, are low in saturated fat, devoid of cholesterol and high in unsaturated fats. But will increasing your consumption of nuts actually decrease your risk of developing cardiovascular disease? It depends. If you replace your mid-afternoon snack of a candy bar with an equivalent number of calories from nuts (there are 160 to 180 in 25 grams), you will be decreasing your intake of saturated fat and *trans*-fatty acids and that's all to the good. But switching from a plain chocolate bar to one with almonds will not likely confer any benefit. And adding nuts without subtracting something else most certainly will not be beneficial, since increased calories will lead to weight gain.

The bottom line: if you enjoy nuts in salads or on yogurt, or plain as a snack, by all means eat them. But when you add nuts to your diet, something else has to come out. Preferably the food you will be eating less of is high in *trans* or saturated fatty acids.

and rapeseed oil and those high in polyunsaturated fatty acids, such as safflower, sunflower and corn oil. It was thought olive oil was particularly beneficial for reducing heart disease risk. However, the scientific evidence no
longer supports that line of thinking. The aim is simply to shoot for more
unsaturated fat and less saturated and *trans* fats. That's the best way of keeping down cholesterol levels.

When it comes to solid rather than liquid fats, go with soft (tub or
spreadable) margarine over butter or hard margarine (unless the label says
it's *trans* fat-free). Or use non-butter blends with little to no saturated fat or
trans-fatty acids per serving. Despite the flak over margarine several years
ago when it was discovered that the *trans*-fatty acids contained in traditional
hard margarine raise LDL-cholesterol as much as the saturated fat found in
butter, there's not much difference between the two. You should limit both.
Generally speaking, the softer and more spreadable the margarine, the less
saturated *and trans* fats it has than other spreads.

Accentuate Whole Grains

GOAL: Four to nine servings daily (at least half from whole grain)

SERVING SIZE: 1 (25g) slice bread

              ½ cup pasta, rice or other cooked grain

              ½ cup cooked oatmeal

              1 serving breakfast cereal (refer to label for serving size)

              ½ sourdough roll

              ½ (50g) bagel

No food component has taken as much of a beating in the public consciousness in the last five years as carbohydrates – the major components of grains.
They have been branded *the* villain of all weight-control efforts.

Well, we have some news for you. It's not true. Carbohydrates are GOOD
FOR YOU! Granted, a recent report from the US Centers for Disease Control and Prevention points to carbohydrate-rich foods as the ones that have
added most of the 300-plus calories daily to the average woman's diet over
the last thirty years. But the bulk of those calories come from *refined* carbohydrates, such as the sugar (high fructose corn syrup) in carbonated drinks

or desserts and the white flour used to make pizza dough and most pasta, salty snacks like pretzels and the refined flour in cakes, biscuits and so on. That is, the problem is not with carbohydrate-rich grains. It's with the particular forms of grains too many of us are eating too much of.

The grains that are heart-healthy are *whole* grains – wholegrain breads and cereals, brown rice and wholewheat pasta. Unlike refined grains, they contain fibre plus a host of nutrients and healthy plant chemicals that are eliminated when grains go through the refining process. No wonder whole grains are the ones that research has shown are associated with decreased heart disease risk in women.

The problem is that wholegrain foods are hard to come by. Only 5 per cent of the packaged grain-based products you'll find in the supermarket are whole grain. And it's not easy to tell which ones they are. Terms such as 'multi grain', 'seven-grain' and 'unbleached flour' on food labels for breads, scones, waffles and the like all sound as though the product is whole grain. But they don't mean a thing as far as whether a grain is truly whole or not. You have to look past the name on the front of the package to the fine print on the ingredients list. If the word 'whole' is part of the first ingredient listed, the food contains whole grain. If not, leave it on the shelf and look for something else. If the label says '100% whole grain' or 'whole wheat', so much the better.

Pretty much the only exceptions in packaged foods are oats and rice. Oats are automatically a whole grain. They are not stripped of their wholegrain components, even if the word 'whole' does not appear on the packaging. And if the rice is *brown* rice, the whole rice grain is in the package. It hasn't gone through the refining process.

Fortunately, there are other wholegrain options besides breads, cereals, rice and related products. One is popcorn. Yes, popcorn; corn is a whole grain. Just make sure it's air-popped rather than made with butter or partially hydrogenated fat (*trans*-fatty acids).

There are also whole grains that you can cook up as starches either for side dishes or for breakfast. For instance, wheatberries are a whole grain that Miriam turns into one of her favourite morning meals (see recipe at the end of this chapter). There's also bulgur, buckwheat groats (kasha), barley, millet, spelt, faro and quinoa (pronounced KEEN-wah). These grains can be served

Salt Shakedown

The amount of salt or, more specifically, sodium in your diet is related to your blood pressure. The more salt you consume each day, the higher your blood pressure is going to be. That said, we all differ in our response to salt; some women's blood pressure is going to drop much more than others' in response to a decline in salt consumption. Still, eating less salt is certainly not harmful and most likely will be beneficial, especially as you age. Most people become more 'salt sensitive' as they get older, with a bigger change in blood pressure depending on the amount of salt they eat.

What's the best way to reduce your salt intake? The vast majority of the salt we eat, as much as 80 per cent, comes from prepared foods. If you follow our advice in this chapter and eat a diet that is predominantly composed of unprocessed foods, you will have more control of your salt intake. There are also some simple rules to follow:

- Don't add salt to your food until you taste it to make certain it really needs it.
- Don't put a salt shaker on the table.
- Don't use salt directly out of the package you buy it in, even for cooking. Transfer some to a shaker so that it is easier to control the amount you add to the food you are preparing.
- If you can see grains of salt on a product, look for one with less.

Many products are now available in 'reduced salt' or 'low-sodium' versions. Try them, especially if you are using them for cooking. You can always add salt, whereas you can't take it out.

Keep in mind that we can 'unlearn' our taste for salt. Our love of sugar is inborn. With salt, within months of cutting back, what was once 'salty enough' will become 'too salty'. Try it and see.

plain and can take the place of brown rice or pasta. Just check the package or a cookbook for preparation instructions.

Whole grains are always available in health food shops but can also be found in many traditional supermarkets, either with the regular items, such as brown rice and wholewheat pasta, or in the 'health foods' section.

We are not saying that every single carbohydrate-rich food you eat has to be a whole grain. But the more, the better – *at least half.* Bear in mind that a lot of grain-based foods contain several servings at once. A 150g bagel from a coffee shop equals five servings from the grains group, not one. Two cups of pasta at an Italian restaurant count as four servings of grains, since a single serving is a half cup. Granted, if that is the centrepiece of the meal, it might be perfectly appropriate to eat several servings at once. What is important is to be aware of it and factor it into your daily food pattern.

Revere Low- and Non-fat Dairy Foods

GOAL: two to three servings daily

SERVING SIZE: 1 cup non-fat or 1% milk

1 cup low- or non-fat yogurt

25g hard cheese (Cheddar, Swiss, etc.)

40g reduced-fat hard cheese

½ cup part-skim ricotta cheese

½ cup non-fat or 1% fat cottage cheese

As every woman knows, dairy products are associated with stronger bones and may keep down blood pressure. All are excellent sources of protein as well as outstanding sources of calcium and other nutrients. It is important to choose low- and non-fat dairy foods to keep saturated fat intake low. (Most are now available in low-lactose varieties, for those who need them.) Combined with other foods, they can really liven things up. (Think a bit of piquant cheese on vegetables or a dollop of yogurt topping a fruit salad.)

But more than three out of four women don't eat enough dairy foods to ensure proper intake of calcium and all the other nutrients dairy provides. We urge you to shoot for *three servings of low- or non-fat dairy foods daily.* It doesn't just have to be a glass of skim or 1 per cent milk or some milk in your cereal. Grate some hard cheese, such as Swiss, Cheddar or Muenster, over the top of a casserole. (If you don't buy reduced-fat hard cheese, you'll want to make especially sure to use cheese as a condiment or to accent a dish rather than as a meal centrepiece because while it's high in calcium and other minerals and vitamins, it's also high in saturated fat.) Or sprinkle plain yogurt with muesli and sunflower or pumpkin seeds or mix it with fresh or frozen fruit.

You can also mix into yogurt dried cherries, sultanas, dried cranberries or any other dried fruit that suits your fancy (for wonderful flavour and texture, mix it in the night before). And mozzarella balls, which have a long refrigerator life, are great for snacks and travel well.

Finally, sandwiches made with low-fat cheese are helped along with some fine mustard and thick slices of ripe tomato.

Target Heart-Healthy Proteins

GOAL: three to four servings daily

SERVING SIZE: 85g cooked fish

½ cup cooked beans

½ cup tofu

1 egg

2 tablespoons peanut butter

85g cooked, skinless poultry

85g cooked lean beef, pork or lamb

By heart-healthy proteins, we mean proteins that don't come coupled with a lot of saturated fat, which some sources of protein do, including fatty cuts of meat and full-fat dairy products.

High on our list of good-for-your-heart proteins is fish. You can certainly follow a heart-healthy eating plan without eating any fish, but if you're not a vegetarian, we urge you to eat *at least two fish meals a week*. The evidence is overwhelming that including some fish in the diet helps stave off heart disease. Of course, fish that are rich in omega-3 fatty acids, including salmon (wild *or* farmed), mackerel and herring, are particularly good for your heart (they tend to have darker-coloured flesh). But we don't want you to get hung up on the type of fish you eat. It's more important, especially if you're not a fish eater currently, simply to begin to incorporate more fish into your diet. Even tuna sandwiches count – but frozen fish fingers, fried clams and fried, breaded shrimp do not. With those choices, the actual amount of fish tends to be rather meagre and the type of cooking fat used tends to be high in *trans-* or saturated fatty acids. The cooking method should keep fat and salt on the relatively low side. The best bets are baked or grilled fish. Not only will they be heart-healthy, but they will also be replacing heart-*un*healthy choices you may have otherwise opted for, say, pasta in cream sauce or a hamburger.

Dr Lichtenstein Talks Safe Fish

You may have read or heard news reports that some types of fish are high in mercury and contaminants called PCBs. But it's not as dangerous as it may sound. In the US, the Food and Drug Administration has issued specific guidelines for only four types of fish: shark, swordfish, king mackerel and tilefish. Furthermore, the advisory caution for these rarely eaten fish is only for women of childbearing years as well as young children. Those groups should not eat any fish from those species. They can eat up to 350g a week – four to six servings – of any other fish except canned white albacore tuna. It has more mercury than canned light tuna, so women of childbearing age and children should eat no more than one 175g can of white albacore a week.

For all other people, there are no fish species that are off limits. Vary the type of fish you eat, as your taste dictates.

As you consider fish, keep in mind the risk/benefit ratio. Your risk of developing cardiovascular disease is relatively high in the scheme of things and the evidence is quite consistent that eating fish on a regular basis reduces that risk. Your risk of mercury toxicity or toxicity of other contaminants, on the other hand, is quite low. When put into perspective, the choice to include fish in the diet doesn't require too much thought.

For specific questions regarding the safety of eating different fish, go to www.food.gov.uk – the UK Foods Standards Agency website.

We want to point out here that even the staunchest non-fish eater can be converted. Alice's teenage daughter turned up her nose at fish until one of her friends brought a tuna sandwich to school with just a little bit of mayo, plenty of curry and a few raisins. She liked it so much that the 'no fish' barrier was broken. Now she will even eat flounder. So experiment for yourself and your family.

Beans are a great protein source, too. They're one of the few protein sources, in fact, that contain a lot of fibre – up to 8g per half cup. And they

To Eat Eggs or Not?

A lot of people think eggs are *verboten* if you're trying to protect your heart. They're not. Yes, they are high in dietary cholesterol. But as we said in chapter 4, we now know that while the cholesterol in food can raise blood cholesterol, saturated fat and *trans*-fatty acids generally raise blood cholesterol – and heart disease risk – considerably more. The amount of cholesterol in your food doesn't correlate with the amount of cholesterol in your bloodstream.

We don't mean that limiting dietary cholesterol isn't important. Both the US National Heart, Lung and Blood Institute's National Cholesterol Education Program and the American Heart Association advise that one limits dietary cholesterol to an average of 300 milligrams a day for healthy people (200 milligrams if you already have heart disease).

An egg yolk (where all the cholesterol resides in an egg) has about 215 milligrams. Meat, fish and full-fat dairy foods have some cholesterol, too. Eight-five grams of cooked chicken, for instance, contains some 65 milligrams and 25g of Swiss cheese has 26. So you have to be thoughtful if you want to eat an egg every single day and stay within the 300-milligram limit. But certainly, you could fit in several eggs a week and not exceed the recommendations. For a lower-cholesterol option, you can substitute two egg whites for one whole egg or use the egg substitutes that are available in the supermarket freezer section.

contain virtually no saturated fat! Always keep a large variety of canned beans in the store cupboard so that you can use them creatively at mealtimes. Throw them into tossed salads, add to vegetable stir-fries and to your favourite soup or simply have them as a side dish.

Beef, pork and chicken are fine on our heart-healthy plan, too, especially if you grill or barbecue them because those methods don't add more calories or saturated fat. Just be sure to keep meat portions on the small side. (If you

Savour a Little Alcohol?

Moderate alcohol consumption – which for women is no more than one drink a day – seems to be protective against heart disease. And it doesn't have to be an 85 to 150ml glass of red wine. It can be white wine, or a 350ml beer or a drink made with 30–45ml of spirits. Red wine does contain phenols, compounds that come from the skin of grapes that have been touted to benefit the heart. But it's the alcohol itself that studies have most consistently linked to a reduced risk for heart disease.

Having said that, we want to make clear that we don't encourage anyone who does not drink to *take up* drinking for the purpose of reducing cardiovascular disease risk. The combined evidence for an eating plan with plenty of vegetables, fruits and whole grains along with some fish, other heart-healthy protein foods and low-fat dairy items is much stronger than the evidence for alcohol, which for some people can be addictive. Moreover, even moderate alcohol intake has been associated with an increased risk of breast cancer – something women at high risk for that disease need to take into consideration when deciding whether to drink. Furthermore, if a woman of child-bearing years becomes pregnant and continues to drink, harm to the foetus may occur.

Finally, it needs to be taken into consideration that a glass of wine, a drink made with spirits or a beer contains anywhere from 100 to 200 calories. That, combined with the potential for alcohol abuse (it's not just a man's problem), should give further pause.

have 175g of chicken, that's two protein servings.) And when it comes to meat, look for lean cuts – generally, ones that have the words 'round' or 'loin' in their names. Those are the cuts that tend to be lower in saturated fat. To keep down saturated fat in *minced* beef, buy at least 93 per cent lean (although no store-bought minced beef is truly very lean, even though the numbers might suggest otherwise).

One way to stretch meat or chicken is with a stir-fry. Neither of us normally uses a recipe. Try the following: sauté a little sliced onion in vegetable oil. When soft (but not brown), add thinly sliced pieces of meat. When the pink is gone, scoop out the meat and add thinly sliced vegetables to the pan – anything from courgettes and peppers to mange-tout, green beans, mushrooms and cauliflower or broccoli florets. Sauté the vegetables until they're wilted. Add the meat back in, stir to heat through again and serve over brown rice.

This same stir-fry template works for extra-firm tofu, high in protein but virtually devoid of saturated fat. The smallish chunks of tofu you cut from a block should brown on the outside edges before you scoop them up from the pan.

Another delicious way to use tofu is to put it in the food processor with sesame seed paste, lemon juice and cumin to taste. If you use silken (rather than firm) tofu, it makes a great vegetable dip, salad dressing or spread.

BRINGING THE 'HEART' ACRONYM TO YOUR TABLE

We believe very strongly that each woman needs to tailor a heart-healthy pattern of eating to her own tastes. But sometimes it's hard to get started. You can know everything you're supposed to do but still have a hard time putting it all together. Hence, the sample eating plan below. It will give you a feel for how all the research comes together to form a heart-healthy dietary pattern.

The plan below will also help you turn on the 'switch' in your head that will allow you to move forward with better eating. Behaviour change can be hard, but with a template that you can tailor to your own preferences, you're one step closer to your heart-healthy eating goal.

Each day's worth of food ranges from about 1,400 to 1,700 calories, including a mandatory fruit snack. If you choose an additional snack or two, it ranges up to 2,000 calories. (Of course, if you want a larger portion at a meal, cut down somewhere else during the day or perhaps on the snacks.) You can mix and match breakfasts, lunches and dinners as you see fit. There isn't any magic to the order in which they are presented because it's never about one or another particular food. It's the overall pattern that makes the difference. Also, this is not a weight-loss plan. If you need to lose weight, you will need to pay particular attention to the serving sizes and opt for fewer snacks (and carefully review chapter 7).

BREAKFAST

Option 1: 'Pick and Choose'   Amount

GRAIN (TWO OF THE FOLLOWING OR A DOUBLE SERVING)

wholegrain cold cereal (see package for serving size)	½ to 1 cup
wholegrain hot cereal (oatmeal, kasha, wheatberries, etc.)	½ cup
wholegrain bread (toasted or plain)	1 (25g) slice
wholegrain bagel or sourdough roll	25g

FRUIT (ONE OF THE FOLLOWING – FRESH, FROZEN OR CANNED)

Whole, fresh fruit (apple, peach, banana, orange, etc.)	1 medium
Whole, fresh fruit (berries, grapes, etc.)	1 cup
Sliced or chopped fruit (melon, peach, etc.)	1 cup fresh or ½ cup frozen
Dried fruit (apricots, prunes, cranberries, etc.)	¼ cup
100% juice	175ml

DAIRY (ONE OF THE FOLLOWING)

Milk (skim or 1%)	225ml
Yogurt (low- or non-fat)	175–225g
Hard cheese (Cheddar, Swiss, etc.)	25g

Low-fat hard cheese	40g
Ricotta cheese (part-skim)	½ cup
Cottage cheese (1% fat or non-fat)	½ cup

Option 2: 'Egg Breakfast'

Omelette (in nonstick pan with vegetable oil spray)	3 egg whites or equivalent egg substitute
Vegetables (sautéed in 1 teaspoon vegetable oil)	½ cup
wholegrain toast (or other grain from above)	1 (25g) slice
One dairy from above	
One fruit from above	

Breakfast: 300 to 400 calories

LUNCH

Option 1: 'Classic Sandwich'   Amount

Wholegrain bread	2 (25g) slices
Lean protein (fish, chicken, turkey, beef)	55g
Vegetables (whatever you prefer)	115g
Mayonnaise (reduced fat) and/or mustard	1 tablespoon
One dairy from above	

Note: If you prefer to have two portions of lean protein in your sandwich, omit the dairy; if you prefer to have two portions of dairy, omit the lean protein.

Option 2: 'Hearty Soup'

Hearty soup (non-cream-based vegetable with beans or meat, such as minestrone)	350ml
Wholewheat bread (pitta or equivalent)	1 to 2 (25g) portions
One dairy from above	

Option 3: 'Zesty Salad'

Lettuce greens (variety)	2 cups
Fish, chicken, cheese or tofu (minimally processed)	55g fish or chicken, 25g cheese, ½ cup tofu
Vegetables (variety, chopped)	½ to 1 cup
Dressing (vegetable oil based)	2 tablespoons
Wholewheat bread (pitta or equivalent)	1 (25g) portion
One dairy from above	

Note: If you prefer to have two portions of lean protein in your salad, omit the dairy; if you prefer to have two portions of dairy, omit the lean protein.

FRUIT
All three lunch options include a fruit serving (see page 81 for serving sizes).

Lunch: 500 to 600 calories

SNACK

To make your diet nutritionally complete, you should include a fruit as a snack at least once during the day (see page 81 for serving sizes).

DINNER

Option 1: 'Traditional'	Amount
Lean meat (fish, chicken, beef, pork, lamb), baked, grilled or poached	85g
Sauce (barbeque, teriyaki, etc.), optional	2 tablespoons
STARCH (CHOOSE ONE FROM BELOW)	
Rice (preferably brown)	½ cup
Pasta (preferably whole wheat)	½ cup

Other whole grain (wheatberries, kasha, barley, etc.)	½ cup
Potato (with 2 tablespoons light sour cream)	1 small
Vegetables (sautéed, grilled, roasted with 1 teaspoon vegetable oil)	½ to 1 cup
Tossed salad (mixture of lettuce and other vegetables)	2 cups
Dressing (vegetable oil based)	2 tablespoons

Option 2: 'One Dish'

Vegetable lasagna (with part-skim ricotta cheese)	7.5x10cm rectangle

(Or any other one-dish meal such as: baked pasta mixed with sautéed vegetables and topped with part-skim mozzarella cheese; or taco with chicken, vegetables and shredded low-fat Cheddar cheese. Serving size no greater than 7.5x10cm rectangle.)

Tossed salad (mixture of lettuce and other vegetables)	2 cups
Dressing (vegetable oil based)	2 tablespoons

Option 3: 'Vegan'

Tofu (extra-firm) or veggie burger	½ cup or 1 burger
Green leafy vegetable (spinach, kale, broccoli, etc.)	½ cup
Rice (brown)	½ cup
Beans (kidney, black, etc.)	½ cup
Tossed salad (mixture of lettuce and other vegetables)	2 cups
Dressing (vegetable oil based)	2 tablespoons

Dinner: 500 to 600 calories

A NOTE ABOUT CALORIES

Calorie ranges for three meals and a mandatory snack, using the tight portion sizes noted above, is 1,400 to 1,700 calories. The reality is there tends to be some drift upward in portion sizes and ingredient variations that can add calories. Thus, the most likely scenario is that this eating pattern will put you closer to 1,700 calories a day rather than 1,400. Everybody's calorie needs are different; therefore, you may find that you need to adjust the serving sizes.

ADDITIONAL SNACK IDEAS

Depending upon your calorie needs, you may be having more than just the single mandatory snack each day. If so, choose from the list below.

Snack Options	Amount
Baby carrots or other raw vegetable with optional dip (see recipe)	10 baby carrots or ½ cup raw vegetables and 2–4 tablespoons dip
Yogurt or milk (non-fat, non-sweetened)	175–225g
Hard cheese	25g
Low-fat hard cheese	40g
Nuts (dry, raw or roasted, low-sodium)	3 tablespoons
Fruit (without added sugar)	1 small to medium or ½ cup frozen or canned, or 1 cup fresh

Each snack provides roughly 80 to 120 calories.

Coffee or tea are okay at each meal with skim or 1% milk and no more than 1 teaspoon of sugar *or* artificial sweetener.

Where Do Treats Fit In?

You may have noticed that we did not include in the food choices any ice cream, cake, biscuits, crisps and so on. We do not mean to say that you

Portion Primer

We cannot stress enough how important it is to be aware of portion sizes. Portion sizes in the United States, for example, have increased greatly in the last thirty years. Even plates in restaurants are bigger, as are cup holders in cars; eating (and drinking!) more and more over time is a very insidious process.

Most people aren't accustomed to thinking carefully enough about portions, even though they know that portion size counts. It's all too simple to forget that a dash of light cream in coffee can easily become 3 tablespoons at 20 calories each; or that a drizzle of maple syrup on pancakes becomes 4 tablespoons or more than 200 calories' worth. Similarly, a pasta meal with breadsticks at an Italian restaurant can easily contain enough grain servings to feed four.

You can balance this – without becoming obsessive. You just need to reeducate yourself about what a proper portion is. Some seem ridiculously small. But that is because they are simply units of measurement, not necessarily amounts that you might normally eat in one sitting.

In this chapter we give the portion sizes for the various food categories. We urge you to measure and weigh your food for a couple of weeks to familiarize yourself with them. Use (and buy if you don't yet have them) a set of measuring spoons and cups and a food scale. What seems like 85g of chicken breast could easily be 175g and what seems like a 40-calorie teaspoon of cooking oil could easily be a 180-calorie tablespoon and a half. The same goes for a half cup of cooked rice or spaghetti. Volume piles on fast. As for baked goods, look at the label or use a scale. Most rolls, bagels and even many slices of bread are larger than 25g. Measure what you normally eat. Once you develop an eye for size, volume and weight, you won't have to keep measuring. You'll know automatically how much breakfast cereal is a serving, how much meat is a 85g portion and so on. It doesn't mean that you can never have two or more portions at once. You can, as long as you don't go over the recommended daily total.

Every six months or so, do a reality check with your measuring utensils. You'd be amazed at how easy it is to drift upward again when you think portion sizes are staying the same.

should never eat them. But, just like when we were kids, they do not have to be on the menu seven days a week. A biscuit or two a couple of times a week is fine. A half cup of ice cream occasionally – also no problem. It's when sweets and salty snacks start to become part of the dietary pattern rather than the exception that a heart-healthy diet veers too far off course.

Portion size is a concern here, too. Try to keep portion sizes of treats on the modest side. Use whatever strategy works. Some people keep mini candy bars in the house and are able to limit themselves to one. Others can keep it to one or two biscuits at a time. If 'in the house' is too close, treat yourself to a frozen yogurt at an ice cream shop once in a while so that you don't always have it tempting you from the kitchen freezer.

SEVEN STRONG HEARTS MENUS

You can actually create any number of menus that suit your fancy from the breakfast, lunch, dinner and snack options we have suggested. However you use these items, the pattern will be right. What follows are merely suggestions. Use them, tweak them or ignore them as you see fit – as long as you make sure to choose from the patterns we recommend above, always staying within portion-size guidelines, especially if weight control is a concern.

⊙ *WELCOMING SPRING* ⊙

Breakfast
Yogurt (plain, non-fat) topped with low-sugar muesli spiked with
sunflower and pumpkin seeds and dried chopped apricots
Navel orange

Lunch
Hearty tossed salad with sliced grilled chicken
Oil and vinegar
Wholewheat pitta with tomato and mustard with slice of Cheddar cheese
Ripe pear

Afternoon snack
Fresh strawberries

Dinner
Tossed green salad
Citrus-Grilled Salmon (see recipe)
Fusilli pasta with a dash of olive oil and garlic and
freshly grated Parmesan cheese
Steamed asparagus

Optional second and third snacks; see snack list for suggestions.

⊙ *SUMMER VACATION* ⊙

Breakfast
Bran flakes topped with milk
Fresh blueberries

Lunch
Curried Tuna Salad Sandwich with lettuce (see recipe)
Wholewheat pitta
Wedge of watermelon

Afternoon Snack
Fresh raspberries and vanilla yogurt

Dinner
Garden salad
Barbecued chicken breast
Small baked potato topped with light sour cream and sprinkle of chives
Grilled courgettes brushed with olive oil

Optional second and third snacks; see snack list for suggestions.

◉ EMBRACING AUTUMN◉

Breakfast
Toasted wholegrain sourdough roll topped with 1% cottage cheese
Half grapefruit

Lunch
Black Bean Salad with Tomato, Avocado and Lime Dressing (see recipe)
Crusty French bread
Ripe peach

Afternoon Snack
Cox's apple

Dinner
Fresh spinach, tomato and part-skim milk mozzarella salad
Roasted turkey breast
Roasted root vegetables (carrots, turnips, sweet potato)
drizzled with balsamic vinegar

Optional second and third snacks; see snack list for suggestions.

○ CELEBRATING WINTER ○

Breakfast
Steel-cut oatmeal with dried fruit
Low- or non-fat milk
Half grapefruit

Lunch
Hearty chicken, barley and vegetable soup
Crusty Tuscan wholewheat bread with Danish Tilsit cheese
Clementine

Afternoon Snack
Gala apple

Dinner
Tossed salad with balsamic vinaigrette dressing
Grilled lean sirloin steak
Wheatberry Salad (see recipe)
Roasted Brussels sprouts with onions

Optional second and third snacks; see snack list for suggestions.

○ WEEKEND FARE ○

Breakfast
Vegetable and cheese omelette
Wholewheat toast
Freshly squeezed orange juice

Lunch
Caesar salad with grated Parmesan cheese
Rye crispbread
Plum

Afternoon Snack
Pineapple

Dinner
Tossed salad
Baked Flounder with Lemon Sauce (see recipe)
Rice pilaf
Steamed carrots and green beans

Optional second and third snacks; see snack list for suggestions.

○ A VEGETARIAN AFFAIR ○

Breakfast
Muesli with dried fruit and nuts
Low- or non-fat milk or soya milk

Lunch
Lentil soup
Wholewheat bread with Swiss cheese, shredded lettuce and zesty mustard
Tomato and cucumber salad with olive oil
Red grapes

Afternoon snack
Honeydew melon and cantaloupe

Dinner
Tossed summer salad with vinaigrette dressing
Vegetable tofu stir-fry with seasonal vegetables
Brown rice
Black beans

Optional second and third snacks; see snack list for suggestions.

◉ *WEEKDAY FARE* ◉

Breakfast
Puffed-wheat cereal with skimmed milk
Blueberries and strawberries

Lunch
Mixed green salad with sliced chicken breast, vegetables, feta cheese,
olives, cherry tomatoes and vinaigrette dressing
Wholewheat pitta
Nectarine

Afternoon Snack
Fruit smoothie with non-fat yogurt

Dinner
Shrimp and vegetable stir-fry (mange-tout, onions,
garlic, mushrooms and peppers)
Wholewheat couscous

Optional second and third snacks; see snack list for suggestions.

STRONG WOMEN, STRONG HEARTS RECIPES

All the recipes listed below, which go with many of the menus you might
want to create, are ones we both use – and love. (If we don't like it, we don't
eat it – and we suggest you follow that guideline, too.)

Citrus-Grilled Salmon

(Four servings)

This is a simple yet delicious way to prepare heart-healthy salmon.

Nonstick cooking spray or 1 tablespoon olive oil
2 lemons
2 limes
4 cloves garlic
Freshly ground pepper (to taste)
450g salmon fillets

Heat the grill to medium-high. Spray a large piece of aluminium foil with nonstick cooking spray and turn it up along the edges. Cut the lemons and limes in half and squeeze all of the juice into a large measuring cup, being careful to strain off any seeds. Peel and chop the garlic. Then whisk the juice, garlic and pepper together. Pour about one-quarter of the mixture into the aluminium foil; place the fish on top and pour the rest of the liquid over the fish. Loosely wrap it up, folding over the foil to keep the moisture in while grilling but with enough openings for the juice to (mostly) evaporate. Grill for about 5 minutes on one side and then open the foil to turn the fish once and continue cooking for a total of 10 to 15 minutes until cooked through (time will vary, depending on grill temperature and thickness of the fish). Cut into four pieces.

BAKED FLOUNDER
WITH LEMON SAUCE

◆

(Four servings)

Here is a quick way to dress up a mild fish.

2 tablespoons low-fat plain yogurt
2 tablespoons reduced-fat mayonnaise
1 tablespoon lemon juice
Fresh dill, chopped
450g flounder fillet

Preheat the oven to 200°C. Mix the yogurt, mayonnaise, lemon juice and dill together. Spread this sauce over the flounder fillet. Bake for about 10 minutes or until fish flakes easily. Take care not to overcook.

CURRIED TUNA

◆

(Two servings)

This is Alice's daughter's favourite recipe for tuna. It is quick and delicious.

One 175g can tuna (packed in water), drained
1 tablespoon reduced-fat mayonnaise
1 teaspoon curry powder or to taste
3 tablespoons raisins
3 tablespoons slivered almonds

Break up the tuna pieces with a fork, mix in the mayonnaise, add the remaining ingredients and toss together.

Variation: Add one medium-sized diced apple or 1 stick celery, chopped.

Black Bean Salad with Tomato, Avocado and Lime Dressing

(Three to four servings)

This recipe is from Miriam's book Strong Women Eat Well *and was created by her collaborator, Judy Knipe. It is a good, quick recipe that is perfect for ripe avocados. Eat the salad the same day you make it – before the avocado changes colour.*

425g canned black beans
115g red onion, diced
1 small green or red pepper, cored and chopped
½ jalapeño pepper, cored, seeded and finely chopped (optional)
70g cherry tomatoes, quartered
½ ripe avocado, diced
2 tablespoons chopped fresh coriander

Dressing

2 tablespoons fresh lime juice
1 teaspoon sherry vinegar
1 tablespoon extra-virgin olive oil
½ teaspoon ground cumin
Salt to taste
Freshly ground black pepper

Drain the beans, rinse them very briefly under cold running water and drain again. Transfer them to a bowl, add the onion, chopped pepper, jalapeño pepper (if using), tomato, avocado and coriander and toss lightly.

Combine all the dressing ingredients in a small bowl and whisk until well mixed. Add the dressing to the bean mixture and stir gently. Cover the salad with greaseproof paper or cling film and allow the flavours to blend for 1 or 2 hours at room temperature or in the refrigerator. Bring the salad back to room temperature before serving.

WHEATBERRIES WITH DRIED CRANBERRIES AND HONEY-ORANGE DRESSING

(Makes 3½ to 4 cups; serving size ½ cup)

This recipe is also adapted from Miriam's book Strong Women Eat Well. *Her colleague Judy Knipe introduced her to wheatberries with this dish. It is a staple in Miriam's house now. The entire family loves it. The wheatberries cook to a beautiful pale colour and a tender but crunchy texture. The dish is delicious served by itself but can also be served for breakfast topped with yogurt or as an accompaniment to meats, fish and poultry.*

> 1 cup summer (soft) wheatberries
> 115ml orange juice
> 4 teaspoons honey
> 6 tablespoons pine nuts
> ¼ cup dried cranberries, coarsely chopped
> Salt to taste

Pour wheatberries into a heavy, medium-sized saucepan, add water to cover thoroughly and bring to the boil. Cover the pan, turn to the heat to low and simmer the berries, covered, for about 2 hours or until the grain is cooked but still crunchy. (The berries cook faster if you soak them overnight.) Drain the wheatberries and transfer to a bowl. You will have a generous 2½ cups.

Mix together the orange juice and honey. Add the sweetened juice to the wheatberries and toss together with the pine nuts and chopped cranberries. Mix well and taste for salt, which, added in very small amounts, brings out the flavour of the fruit.

Serve warm, at room temperature or cold.

CLASSIC VINAIGRETTE DRESSING

Miriam learned how to prepare this dressing in a cooking class while studying abroad during college.

150ml good-quality olive oil
75ml balsamic vinegar
1 teaspoon dried basil or 1 tablespoon fresh
1 tablespoon French mustard
½ teaspoon sugar
½ teaspoon salt
Freshly ground black pepper to taste

Pour into a salad dressing decanter, insert stopper and shake vigorously.

SUMMER CUCUMBER DIP

(Makes 3 cups; serving size 2 tablespoons)

This dip is the perfect complement for baby carrots, peppers or other vegetables.

½ cucumber
2 cups plain non-fat yogurt
½ teaspoon salt
2 cloves garlic, crushed
1 tablespoon olive oil

Peel, seed and shred the cucumber. In a colander, press the liquid out of the cucumber. Mix the yogurt, salt, garlic and olive oil in a bowl, stir in the cucumber and serve.

CHAPTER 6

The Right Exercises for Optimal Heart Health

As I got older, I wanted to make sure I wasn't going to get heart disease. I also knew that it was going to get harder and harder to maintain my weight. But my exercise had always been episodic; I'm talking four to six times a year.

For me, the logical way to get into it was to join a gym, but I couldn't bring myself to go because I was so incredibly intimidated by all the machines and weights. I was resisting because I was embarrassed and rationalizing that I didn't have time. Finally, I went to the local YWCA. I decided to go on Saturday mornings. I knew I should be doing this several times a week, but you've got to start somewhere.

When I first got there, I was relieved, first of all, because people were in sweatshirts and pants. It wasn't as if they were all wearing Lycra! Also, they were all shapes, sizes and ages. I had thought no gym would ever have people like me – a woman in her fifties who's not a trained athlete and doesn't have a perfect figure. Plus, a trainer spent an entire hour with me, showing me how to use the machines. This was routine. It had never occurred to me that they would do this.

Three years ago, I couldn't have imagined walking into a gym and using any of the machines. I never thought about my 'abs'. I am now 100 per cent committed.

– HELEN

Along with good, wholesome nutrition, there is no more important thing you can do for your heart than move your body – get your heart rate up, use your muscles and expend more energy. But a regular exercise routine does a lot more than protect your heart. It also improves outlook, increases bone density, ups your energy level, retards the muscle atrophy and creeping frailty that occur as we age and is crucial, as you will learn in the next chapter, for weight control. Says Helen, 'I have not gained weight since menopause, as some of my friends have'.

There are two types of physical activity that we encourage you to incorporate into your lifestyle: aerobic activity and strength training. On top of those two kinds of planned exercise, we hope you will engage in something we call *decreasing sedentary living* – using your body to move through the day in a way you might not have been doing until now, especially if you work at a desk job or don't go out much.

Even with the different activities combined, we're only talking about three to six hours a week. We understand that your schedule might already be packed and that you feel you can't possibly see your way to incorporating something new into your calendar. But what we both have heard over and over again is that while a woman might feel tired for the first couple of weeks after she starts an exercise programme, a physical activity regime so enhances a person's energy level and feelings of well-being that she soon doesn't know how she was able to go for so many years *without* regular exercise. As Helen describes it, 'I can walk up five flights of stairs now and not even think about it. I can jog three miles on a treadmill instead of walking a mile or two. It's easier to carry heavy things. I don't get back pain anymore when I sit at the computer.'

Following is a step-by-step plan for making the different prongs of our exercise programme a part of your life. At all points we emphasize *gradual* adaptation to increased physical activity. Try to tackle too much too fast and you'll end up exhausted, achy and uncomfortable. Add to your exercise routine in a slow, deliberate manner and within just a few weeks you will truly start to feel like a new person. Your heart health will benefit almost immediately, too. Within weeks of beginning an exercise programme, blood pressure starts to drop and the heart begins to beat more efficiently. You'll *feel* great, too.

FIRST STEP: DECREASE SEDENTARY LIVING

In the spirit of taking this one sure step at a time, we feel it is very important that before you begin a formal exercise programme, you spend two weeks finding ways in your routine to decrease a sedentary lifestyle. You may want to start by engaging in brisk walking and strength training right away, but we guarantee that if you spend just two weeks taking stock of your current level of physical activity and see where you can unobtrusively 'insert' more here and there – that is, if you begin by raising your level of activity consciousness – you'll be much more prepared to begin the formal programme and you'll be more likely to succeed.

We're talking about things you've heard a lot about but that few people actually do: taking the stairs instead of the lift; not driving around the supermarket parking lot to find the space closest to the entrance but parking instead wherever you first see a space; walking rather than driving to destinations you can reach on foot within ten minutes (which will ensure walking a mile there and back); getting up to turn the television on and off manually rather than using the remote; and so on.

It may not seem like it adds up to much, but it does. You can easily burn an extra 100 calories a day with those small bursts of physical activity – enough to lose 10 excess pounds (4.5 kilos) in a year without eating less. And, of course, every time you move around rather than sit, you challenge your heart to beat a little faster, training it to be stronger and fitter. That is, the more you push your heart and the rest of your cardiovascular system to do, the more they *can* do.

We both engage in exactly the things we're encouraging. It isn't always easy and we aren't perfect all the time, but overall we are pretty consistent. Alice works on the fifth floor of a research centre at Tufts and often walks up to her office rather than taking the lift. And she rarely uses the lift to go from floor to floor once she's in the building. Miriam, too, doesn't use the lift in her eight-story research building a block and a half away. And neither of us wastes time driving around the shopping centre looking for a spot close to the entrance. We also walk or ride our bicycles when we can (Miriam lives one-and-a-half miles from her town centre, Alice, several blocks from her post office) and do not shy away from some of the heavier work around the garden, including digging the flowerbeds or raking leaves.

Obviously, if you have been sedentary for most or all of your adult life, you should not start trying to decrease your sedentariness by digging for a half hour or walking up ten flights of stairs to your office. Not only could it dissolve your resolve to push on even before you truly get started, it could also be risky. But just about all women can think of safe ways to incorporate a little more physical activity into their lives here and there, even if it's as simple as taking something upstairs every time you think of it rather than building a pile at the bottom of the stairs to take up in one trip at the end of the day.

You'll be surprised at the end of two weeks how many little 'pieces' of physical activity you can tuck into your day without losing a lot of time – or energy. You'll be surprised, too, at the sense of self-confidence you begin to enjoy by using your body more. Furthermore, you'll be more ready to tackle the structured part of our exercise plan, both physically and emotionally.

BEFORE YOU START THE FORMAL PROGRAMME

After two weeks of making a concentrated effort to get more physical activity here and there, you might be eager to get the actual exercise sessions under way. Before you do, we strongly advise you to take the PAR-Q (Physical Activity Readiness Questionnaire) that follows.

Nearly everyone can participate in our exercise programme without any problems, but by taking the PAR-Q, you're adding an extra level of caution – never a bad thing. (If you're over 70, the PAR-Q alone will not be enough. We strongly recommend that you see your doctor to get a professional go-ahead before taking up an exercise plan.)

Exercise Clothes, Gear and Personal Effects

You are going to need to buy some essentials to get you going – both correctly and safely. It'll be a pretty modest investment overall – even more so when you consider the return in health benefits.

Athletic Shoes

Last year Miriam trained for the Boston Marathon as part of a large effort at Tufts called the President's Marathon Challenge. Even she, an accomplished athlete, had a hard time finding the right athletic shoes for her training runs – her feet are very narrow. But she kept at it until she tried on a pair that fit comfortably, had the right stability for her gait and were light enough for long-distance running.

Admittedly, training for a marathon is different from incorporating a regular programme of physical activity into your routine, but either way, the comfort and health of your feet are critical for your success. So choose carefully. Make sure the shoe fits – and also fits the type of exercise in which you plan to participate. (For instance, running shoes tend to be lighter than walking shoes.) And once your athletic shoes are six to nine months old, consider buying a new pair. To check whether your shoes are worn out, place them on a table or counter at eye level and look to see whether the soles are worn on either the outside or the inside edges. That should be the trigger that sends you back to a store where the salespeople have expertise in fitting shoes. Exercising with shoes that are worn out puts too much stress on the joints. That's true for *all* your shoes, not just the ones you work out in.

Dumbbells

Unless you join a fitness centre you will need to buy some dumbbells. The strength-training component of the programme requires starting with a 1.5kg (3lb) and a 2.5kg (5lb) pair of dumbbells or hand weights. As you get stronger, you will need pairs of 3kg, 4kg, 4.5kg (6, 8, 10) and, in some cases, 5.5kg (12lb) dumbbells, available at sporting good stores and many department stores. (But you can wait until you get to that level to buy those.) Prices start at around £10 per pair. Some dumbbells are adjustable by weight so you don't have to buy more than one pair. If you go that route, make sure they are comfortable to hold – and easy to adjust.

Staircase, Step or Utility Stool

One of the exercises requires a step. You need to buy a step or stool *only* if you don't have a staircase at home. You can buy a step for about £25 at a sporting goods shop – or a sturdy utility stool 20–30cm (8–12in) high for £5

Physical Activity Readiness
Questionnare – PAR-Q
(revised 1994)

PAR-Q & YOU

(A Questionnaire for People Aged 15 to 69)

Regular physical activity is fun and healthy and increasingly more people are starting to become more active every day. Being more active is very safe for most people. However, some people should check with their doctor before they start becoming much more physically active.

If you are planning to become much more physically active than you are now, start by answering the seven questions in the box below. If you are between the ages of 15 and 69, the PAR-Q will tell you if you should check with your doctor before you start. If you are over 69 years of age and you are not used to being very active, check with your doctor.

Common sense is your best guide when you answer these questions. Please read the questions carefully and answer each one honestly: check YES or NO.

YES	NO	
☐	☐	1. Has your doctor ever said that you have a heart condition *and* that you should only do physical activity recommended by a doctor?
☐	☐	2. Do you feel pain in your chest when you do physical activity?
☐	☐	3. In the past month, have you had chest pain when you were not doing physical activity?
☐	☐	4. Do you lose your balance because of dizziness or do you ever lose consciousness?
☐	☐	5. Do you have a bone or joint problem that could be made worse by a change in your physical activity?
☐	☐	6. Is your doctor currently prescribing drugs for your blood pressure or heart condition?
☐	☐	7. Do you know of *any other reason* why you should not do physical activity?

IF
YOU
ANSWERED

YES to one or more questions

Talk with your doctor by phone or in person BEFORE you start becoming much more physically active or BEFORE you have a fitness appraisal. Tell your doctor about the PAR-Q and which questions you answered YES.

- You may be able to do any activity you want – as long as you start slowly and build up gradually. Or, you may need to restrict your activities to those which are safe for you. Talk with your doctor about the kinds of activities you wish to participate in and follow his/her advice.
- Find out which community programmes are safe and helpful for you.

NO to all questions

If you answered NO honestly to <u>all</u> PAR-Q questions, you can be reasonably sure that you can:

- start becoming much more physically active – begin slowly and build up gradually. This is the safest and easiest way to go.
- take part in a fitness appraisal – this is an excellent way to determine your basic fitness so that you can plan the best way for you to live actively.

➡

DELAY BECOMING MUCH MORE ACTIVE:

- if you are not feeling well because of a temporary illness such as a cold or fever – wait until you feel better; or
- if you are or may be pregnant – talk to your doctor before you start becoming more active.

Please note: If your health changes so that you then answer YES to any of the above questions, tell your fitness trainer or health professional. Ask whether you should change your physical activity plan.

Informed Use of the PAR-Q: The Canadian Society for Exercise Physiology, Health Canada, agents assume no liability for persons who undertake physical activity and if in doubt after completing this questionnaire, consult your doctor prior to physical activity.

to £10. You should be able to find the stool at a hardware store or a good department store. Make sure the stool has four solid legs and a skid-proof top. Make sure, too, that it can hold your body weight easily without tipping over.

Exercise Mat
It may seem superfluous, but a firm exercise mat makes floor exercises more comfortable. Exercise mats are relatively inexpensive (about £10) and easy to store and they make a real difference. Alternatively, you can use a large bath towel. Either one provides added cushioning.

Tops and Bottoms
Make sure to wear loose, non-restrictive clothing for comfort and to dress appropriately for the weather. (Wear layers in winter so you can tie an outer layer around your waist if you warm up too much as you're going along.)

The newest quick-dry fabrics available for athletic clothing dry quickly when they get wet. It's a big step in improving comfort while you work out. The wetness doesn't turn cold and stick to your body.

You don't need to buy those clothes right now. You most likely have what you need in your wardrobe. As you get more into the programme, you can supplement your workout clothes with what's appropriate. (Or you can drop a nice hint to a friend or family member when your birthday is approaching.)

Sun Protection
Get a hat with a visor to protect your eyes, and sunglasses, too. Also, in summer, always use sunscreen. Keep a small container of sunscreen with your water bottle. That way, you won't forget to use it.

Water
Last year, the US National Academy of Sciences issued a statement saying that it isn't necessary to follow the popular advice to drink at least eight glasses of water a day but, rather, to drink only when you feel thirsty. Nonetheless, we believe water should be an integral part of your workout gear. Drink some just before and just after your aerobic workouts as well as during strength training. Plenty of fluid will allow your body to perform at its best.

Contrary to what you might see in ads, you do not need a sports drink to rehydrate. You don't need the extra calories, either. Sports drinks are for exercise that is of long duration – more than 1½ hours at a time or if you are working out for a long time in the heat. Stick to good old H_2O instead.

THE STRONG WOMEN, STRONG HEARTS EXERCISE PROGRAMME

We put forth here two different possibilities for exercise programmes:

- *Minimal* Heart-Healthy Exercise Programme
- *Optimal* Heart-Healthy Exercise Programme

To produce meaningful results in your cardiovascular system and reduce your risk of heart disease significantly, your level of exercise should fall somewhere on the spectrum between the two programme levels. Minimal is fine, especially as a first step. You get the best from your effort by going from being completely sedentary to moderately active. But the more you do, the better shape your heart will be in.

Minimal Exercise Programme at a Glance

Aerobics:	30 minutes at a time, three days a week, or 15 minutes at a time, six days a week
Flexibility (Stretching):	5 minutes following every exercise session

Optimal Exercise Programme at a Glance

Aerobics:	30 or more minutes at a time, five to six days a week
Strength training:	30 minutes at a time, two to three days a week
Flexibility (Stretching):	5 minutes following every exercise session

For some of you, the programmes may look daunting. You may never have exercised regularly before or it may be a long time since you did. For that reason, we cannot emphasize enough that the key to long-term success is to take it slowly but deliberately. At all points, our programme encourages you to increase the duration and intensity of your exercise *a little bit at a time.* That will keep you from burning out – and injuring yourself. And for the aerobic exercises, in particular, choose exercises that you enjoy. That's also crucial for sticking with the programme.

If you *are* starting from scratch, don't go for thirty minutes of aerobics all at once. Start with short bouts (ten to fifteen minutes in duration) and only half the strength-training routine and work up from there. The most important thing is *consistency*. Don't tell yourself not to bother because you can't do much at the start. Keep building on it little by little, individualizing the programme so that you stay committed and continue to build on what you've accomplished.

No matter what your initial level of activity and how slowly you proceed, in just a couple of weeks your endurance and strength will increase. Within six weeks, added vigour and vitality will kick in.

Most women choose brisk walking because you don't have to go to a gym to do it and because everybody knows how to walk. It's not something you have to learn or get better at. But if you really love swimming or biking or some other form of aerobics, go for it. Or cross-train by doing some brisk walking combined with another aerobic activity.

Cross-training might be best for someone who likes to swim or exercise on a bicycle. Walking and running, unlike swimming and biking, are weight-bearing exercises, meaning you carry the weight of your body as you perform the activity. They have an added advantage in that, unlike activities in which you sit or are carried by water, they help maintain the strength of your bones.

Warming Up and Cooling Down

One last bit of preparation before you begin the actual programme. Most exercise injuries result from the body (muscles and connective tissue, specifically) not being warmed up or cooled down adequately. To warm up and avoid hurting yourself, do three to five minutes of low-intensity walking, dancing, calisthenics or riding a stationary bike before you actually begin the exercise. Many people like to do a milder version of the activity they plan to engage in: walking before running, for instance, or cycling slowly before going at it with greater intensity. A low-intensity warm-up increases muscle and tendon elasticity – the 'rubber bands' of your body will have more give – and that in turn decreases the chances of one of them 'snapping'. Your heart and the rest of your vascular system will also be ready for the workout; they won't have to go into high gear all at once.

A proper cool-down is just as critical for safe exercising. It allows your body to return *slowly* to its resting state. Your heart rate will decrease gradually, as will your blood pressure, easing stress on your system. And, when you cool down properly, the blood in your legs will slowly be shifted back to the rest of your body. Five minutes of light activity – the other 'bookend' around your exercise session – will suffice as a cool-down.

If your exercise session is strength training rather than aerobics, a good cool-down is stretching, which takes care of cooling down and flexibility at the same time.

The Aerobic Component

To get heart-healthy results from aerobic exercise, which directly targets the heart, lungs and the rest of the cardiovascular system, the key is working out at the appropriate *intensity* for a long enough *duration* to make a difference. If you go at it too easily, you won't experience enough improvement. (Going at it too hard can cause injuries and do your heart more harm than good, although

At Home or at the Fitness Centre?

Some people prefer exercising at home because of the convenience, the privacy and the lack of a membership fee. Others prefer having an exercise buddy to keep them motivated. Still others prefer a gym or community centre because they can get instruction and guidance from professionals and also use weights *or* resistance machines to vary their strength-training sessions. Some people are lucky enough to have fitness centres at their places of work. It doesn't matter where you exercise. Just make sure it's a place you feel comfortable. There's no point in joining a gym that's either out of the way or filled with members who make you feel intimidated (although, like Helen, you might be surprised to find that a lot of people joining gyms these days look just like you). You'll just end up talking yourself out of going more times than not.

If it's instruction that you need, another option is to go for a personal trainer at home. They can be expensive – up to £50 an hour – but a few sessions may be all you need to get you started and to ensure you're using the proper form and technique. A personal trainer can also help you become and stay motivated.

that very rarely occurs. The overwhelming majority of people, when they err, err on the side of not pushing themselves hard enough.)

Determining the Right Intensity

When it is working at its hardest, your heart can beat a certain maximum number of beats per minute. But that's too much for regular exercise, even exercise that lasts only a short while. The right intensity, or range, for exercise is generally 60 to 80 per cent of your maximum heart rate. It's safe yet rigorous enough to bring your cardiovascular system to the next level. How do you figure out your maximum heart rate so you can determine 60 to 80 per cent of it? It's simple.

Maximum Heart Rate = 220 Minus Your Age

The equation is not perfect. It doesn't take into account variations from person to person. But it's a reasonable ballpark measure that you can use in conjunction with how you feel as you're going along. In other words, if you're exercising at 80 per cent of your maximum heart rate but feel like you can't get in enough air or keep up the pace, you'll want to take it down a little.

The following chart gives heart rates – beats per minute – for 60, 70, 80 and 90 per cent intensity for a number of ages based on five-year intervals. If your age is not one of the five-year marks, subtract it from 220 and multiply it by 0.60, 0.70, 0.80 or 0.90. That will give you the range of target heart rates for your age.

Target Heart Rate = 60 to 80 per cent of Maximun Heart Rate

	HEART RATE IN BEATS PER MINUTE AT DIFFERENT PER CENTS OF MAXIMUM			
AGE	60%	70%	80%	90%
20	120	140	160	180
25	117	137	156	176
30	114	133	152	171
35	111	130	148	167
40	108	126	144	162
45	105	123	140	158
50	102	119	136	153
55	99	116	132	149
60	96	112	128	144
65	93	109	124	140
70	90	105	120	135
75	87	102	116	131
80	84	98	112	126

Of course, once you learn the range for your target heart rate, you need to be able to determine whether you are in that range while you're actually exercising. There are two ways to do that. One is to take your pulse. The other is to use an intensity scale. Many exercisers use a combination of both.

Taking Your Pulse

To take your pulse, hold out your right hand. Press together the index finger and middle finger of your left hand and touch them to the inside of the base of your wrist, just past where your hand ends. Slide your fingers across your right wrist, pressing firmly when you're at the hollow next to the tendons. If you can't feel your pulse, vary how firmly you're pressing or bend your wrist back slightly. Then, watching a clock with a second hand, count the number of beats for thirty seconds, then multiply by two.

You should check your heart rate when you've been doing aerobic activity for five minutes as well as at the end of your workout session, just before you cool down. That way, you can tell whether you're exercising at a high enough intensity (at least 60 per cent of your maximum heart rate) but not too high (more than 80 per cent).

Note: You don't have to use your fingers to take your pulse. You can buy a heart rate monitor – a strap worn around your mid-chest that sends a signal to a watch on your wrist that gives a heart rate readout. But while heart rate monitors can be useful, they're expensive – £25 to £100, depending on the model.

Using the Intensity Scale

Knowing whether you're in the target heart rate range is the most precise way of determining whether you're doing your aerobic exercise at the appropriate intensity. But once you've been exercising for a while and know what it feels like to be in the effective range (this middle ground entails a certain amount of sweating and laboured breathing), you can rely more often on the intensity scale. It's a five-point scale, with level 3 corresponding to 60 to 80 per cent of your heart rate maximum and occasionally going up to 4.

At level 3, you should more or less be able to keep up a conversation. At level 4, you can complete a couple of sentences here and there. If you can't utter more than a word or two at a time, you're probably exercising at above 90 per cent of your maximum heart rate – an unsafe level.

Note: When it's hot or humid outside, the body has a harder time getting rid of its heat. Therefore, working out at any given intensity can result in heart rates that are 10 to 20 beats higher per minute than usual. Be sure to tone down your activity level a bit to account for this factor.

Don't Overdo

We want your exercise to feel like exercise. But if you have not been doing any aerobic activities, you really want to *start slowly* – maybe just five to ten minutes of an activity at a low intensity. Don't worry about intensity at first. After two or three weeks you can begin to increase it, as well as the time spent exercising. If that feels too drawn out, keep in mind that some people haven't exercised in decades. A few weeks of taking it slow isn't going to make a difference. The point at the beginning is that you've started.

Here's a suggested pattern for increasing your aerobic exercise intensity and duration. Remember, the *minimum* you eventually want to work up to is at least thirty minutes three times a week (or fifteen-minute bouts six times a week). The *optimal* is thirty to sixty minutes five to six times a week.

Week 1	60–70% Maximum Heart Rate	5–10 minutes
Week 2	60–70% Maximum Heart Rate	10 minutes
Week 3	60–70% Maximum Heart Rate	15 minutes
Week 4	60–80% Maximum Heart Rate	15 minutes
Week 5	60–80% Maximum Heart Rate	20 minutes
Week 6 and beyond	60–80% Maximum Heart Rate	30 or more minutes

EXERCISE INTENSITY SCALE FOR AEROBIC TRAINING	
EXERCISE INTENSITY LEVEL	DESCRIPTION OF EFFORT
1. Sedentary	No perceived effort: standing, sitting or lying down.
2. Active This level contributes to overall health and burns more calories than being sedentary.	Easy, sustainable movement that causes a small increase in heart and breathing rate and doesn't raise a sweat (unless the weather is hot): strolling, light gardening, slow dancing, golfing.
3. Moderate training You should exercise at this level to condition your heart and the rest of your cardio-vascular system.	Somewhat hard movement that elevates the heart rate to 60 to 70 per cent of maximum most of the time, ranging up to 80 per cent. Breathing is more rapid, though it's possible to converse with only slightly altered speech; perspiration appears after about 5 to 15 minutes, depending on air temperature.
4. Vigorous training This is a more advanced level of aerobic conditioning that becomes an appropriate goal after exercising for several months.	Hard effort that elevates the heart rate to 70 to 80 per cent most of the time, ranging up to 90 per cent of maximum. Breathing is more rapid but not laboured – it's possible to converse, though faster breathing will cause evident interruptions; perspiration starts within 5 to 10 minutes, depending on air temperature; fatigue increases as the workout continues and you will feel a need to stop by the end.
5. Overexertion Not recommended!	Excessive effort: heart pounds to the point of discomfort or nausea; breathing is too rapid to permit speech.

A Note About Warm-up and Cool-down

You will not be at your target heart rate the entire time you are doing aerobic exercise. It takes about five minutes to work up to it (the warm-up) and five minutes to slow down before you finish in order to ease your muscles out of their more strenuous work (the cool-down). In other words, you do not have to tack on extra time to your aerobics routine for warm-ups and cool-downs. If you exercise for, say, thirty minutes, ten of those minutes will be warm-up and cool-down and twenty will be you working at your target heart rate. That's fine.

That said, it does get a little trickier if you are doing shorter bouts. You will need to add on a little more time to account for the warm-up and cool-down. That's because you need to be at your target heart rate for at least ten minutes at a stretch to truly strengthen your cardiovascular system.

Remember to Enjoy It!

As we said earlier in this chapter, the best aerobic activities are the ones you enjoy, because they're the ones you'll stick with. Most people choose brisk walking, which is great because it can be done just about anywhere with not much more equipment than a good pair of exercise shoes (that are not worn out). Just keep in mind that the walking shouldn't feel like a stroll, even if you go with a friend. Whether on a pavement, in a shopping mall, on hilly terrain or on a treadmill, it should feel purposeful, as if you are pushing yourself to catch a bus or make a meeting on time. That is, by the time you're finished, you should have got warm enough to have broken into at least a light sweat. (It *is* ladylike to sweat. Health, strength, vigour and vitality are all part of being feminine.)

Along with walking, many people enjoy doing their weight-bearing aerobic activity on *cross-country ski machines* and *elliptical trainers*. A lot of women, in particular, also like using *stair climbers* and *stair-stepping* machines. In addition to providing a great workout, they target the legs, buttocks and trunk, which many women want to firm up. Exercise classes ranging from *low-impact aerobics* to *boxing* to *dancing* keep women motivated, too. If you want to dance for exercise – but in privacy – rent or buy a dance exercise video. There are also yoga and tai chi, which we will talk about in greater detail in chapter 8.

Non-weight bearing exercises, as we said earlier, include swimming and biking. (When's the last time you were on a bike? Try it! Just don't forget to

What About a Pedometer?

If you are incorporating more walking into your everyday life as part of your work or errands, etc., pedometers are a great tool for determining whether you are actually getting enough exercise. We highly recommend that you wear one to keep track. Health experts say that optimally, you should be accumulating 10,000 steps each day and we agree. You might not always reach 10,000; it translates to about 4.5 miles (about 7km) over the course of the day. But whether or not you get to that level on a regular basis, a pedometer is a great motivator. Once you have a number, you have a goal – to increase it. Make sure that you follow the manufacturer's directions when wearing the device. Also, keep in mind that you don't need a fancy one. We like the ones that just count steps and nothing more. They cost £10 to £15. See the Resources section for information on purchasing a pedometer.

wear your helmet.) You can also choose rowing – a great whole-body exercise. Non-weight bearing activities are particularly useful at the start for women with osteoarthritis of the knee or hip because they take pressure off the diseased joints in those body parts. But as you progress, do try to incorporate at least some weight-bearing activities in your exercise routine.

THE STRENGTH TRAINING COMPONENT

While aerobic exercise directly targets the heart, lungs and the rest of the cardiovascular system, strength training is crucial to heart health because it enhances the effect through whole-body muscle conditioning. There's also evidence that it lowers blood pressure. And it reduces fat around the abdomen, which lowers heart disease risk, too.

As with aerobic activities, the key to strength training is to do it regularly – and at the right intensity. You want to challenge your muscles to the point that they adapt to handling a greater amount of weight and become stronger. If you lift weights that are too light, your muscles will not be stimulated enough to 'respond'. If you lift weights that are too heavy, you can end up injuring not only your muscles but also the joints and other tissues that surround them.

A key point here – and this differs from aerobic activities – is that you must let your muscles *rest* by not strength-training them two days in a row. For every strength-training day on, a set of muscles has to have *the next day off*. That's why you'll never see a recommendation to strength-train, from us or any other certified health expert, four to seven days a week. The American Heart Association recommends strength training two days a week. We think that's perfectly acceptable, but we prefer the American College of Sports Medicine's recommendation: *two to three* days per week. Consistency trumps frequency, however. Strength training two days a week every single week is much better than three days a week for a couple of weeks, then once a week for a few more weeks, etc.

What exactly is involved in a strength-training session? In the particular programme we outline here, which targets the entire body – trunk, arms and legs – there are six exercises. Every single time you do one of the exercises – whether it's lifting dumbbells over your shoulders or raising your chest off the floor while lying facedown – it's called a repetition, or rep. Twelve reps make a set and you want to do *two sets of each exercise* during each exercise session, with a minute or so of rest between sets.

Determining the Right Strength-Training Intensity

If you can do more than 12 reps easily, you're not challenging your muscles enough. And if you can do only 5 or 6 reps before having to stop, you're pushing your muscles to deal with too much at once. If you're conducting the moves at the right intensity, the weight you're lifting or pushing against should feel moderately heavy as you start (but well within your ability), then feel as if it's getting heavier and heavier by the sixth or seventh rep. By the twelfth rep, which you should still be able to do in good form, you should feel as if you don't stop and take a break, you couldn't do another one.

As with aerobic exercise, we have developed a scale for evaluating the intensity of your effort. You should use it to judge your intensity at the end of two sets of 12 reps.

EXERCISE INTENSITY SCALE FOR STRENGTH TRAINING	
EXERCISE INTENSITY LEVEL	DESCRIPTION OF EFFORT
1 – Very easy	Too easy to be noticed, like lifting a pencil.
2 – Easy	Can be felt but isn't fatiguing, like carrying a book.
3 – Moderate	Fatiguing only if prolonged – like carrying a full handbag that seems heavier as the day goes on.
4 – Hard	More than moderate at first and becoming difficult by the time you complete 6 or 7 repetitions. You can make the effort 12 times in good form but need to rest afterwards. Think of lifting a 2.5kg (5lb) bag of potatoes or 4 litres (a gallon) of water multiple times.
5 – Extremely Hard	Requires all your strength, like lifting a piece of heavy furniture that you can lift only once, if at all.

Working Up Gradually

The ultimate goal is to reach an intensity of 4 for each exercise. But whenever you're trying a new strength-training move for the first time, the intensity should be a 3 or less. You need time to perfect your form and let the muscles get used to each set of moves. After a few workout sessions, it's time to increase the intensity to 4.

To go from a lower to a greater intensity is to work through *progressions*. Progressions will be provided for most of the exercises and everyone should start with the first progression until the form is mastered. And work up from there.

Try to increase progressions every other workout – or every week – for the first couple of months. For instance, if the progression is to increase the amount of weight you lift, increase the weight by one increment, say, going from 2.5kg (5lb) to 3kg (6lb) dumbbells. Of course, as you become stronger, that weight will not seem like so much and the intensity will drop below a 4 again. It's at that point that you should proceed to the next progression and so on. As you progress over time, the intervals at which you do so will become farther and farther apart. Remember, no matter what progression you are at, always perform two sets of 12 repetitions. The number of reps and sets never changes.

You may find that your muscles feel sore after the first few workouts that are a 4 on the intensity scale (a few people get mild soreness the first couple of times regardless of intensity). That's okay. In fact, it's desirable. It's a sign that you are challenging your muscles to an appropriate degree. But the soreness should *not* interfere with your routine activities. If it does, move down one progression for a week or two.

Don't be discouraged if you move through the progressions for some of the exercises faster than for others. Most people start out with some muscles stronger than others, so progressing more quickly with those is bound to happen. Just bear in mind that *all* of your muscle groups will become stronger if you keep at it. As with aerobic exercise, beginning slowly and progressing gradually but consistently is what works over the long run.

Before You Begin

For safety's sake, you'll need to warm up before you strength-train, just as you do with aerobic activity, with three to five minutes of light activity. You can take a brisk walk around the block or just march in place, but do something with your body before you start lifting. Cool-down for strength training will consist of the stretching exercises described in the Flexibility section later in this chapter.

Tempo and Form

With strength training, the timing of each repetition is everything and that timing is rather slow. You want to make sure it's your muscles that are doing the work – not gravity and not momentum. To that end, a single lift should take about eight seconds: three to raise the weight, a one-second pause and four to return to the starting position. Then pause again while you take a breath before starting the next rep. *Never rush your strength training.*

After you have finished a set of reps, rest from 30 seconds to a minute before starting the second set. Resting is not wasting time. That short time interval increases blood flow and nutrients to the muscles and washes away metabolic waste.

For each exercise, there is a correct form. That's how you ensure that you're targeting, or isolating, the right muscles. It is important to actually *visualize* these muscles contracting to lift and stretching while returning to the starting position. The best way to work it is *not* to tense up the other muscles in your body as you're tensing the ones meant to be used for the lift. Use the brief pause after lifting to scan your body for tension in areas other than the muscles you're trying to work – and relax them. These are a couple of areas that commonly tense up when people exercise:

Face: Don't furrow or knit your brow. And don't clench your teeth or tighten your jaw.

Shoulders: Don't scrunch your shoulders up towards your ears. Don't push them forward, either, which only serves to round the chest and keep you from taking full, deep breaths. Keep your shoulders down and back – relaxed. That will relieve tension in your neck, too.

Posture: Along with keeping your shoulders relaxed, keep your chin tucked in, your abdominal muscles firm and your back straight but relaxed (not arched).

Breathe!
Also important is breathing throughout the exercises. *Never hold your breath.* That can raise blood pressure as you lift the weight, reducing the blood flow to your muscles.

Exhale as you lift the weight and inhale as you lower it. It is counter-intuitive to what you might do naturally, but that's the right way to go. Don't worry if you can't get the right rhythm when you first start. Just keep breathing. As you become more comfortable with the whole process, you'll be able to incorporate the breathing rhythm correctly.

We have found that it really helps people new to strength training to count out loud the eight seconds of each rep. That facilitates breathing *and* doing the exercises at the appropriate tempo.

Make It Your Own

If you do the following exercises twice a week, you'll be doing a lot to get your cardiovascular system – and the rest of your body – in great shape. If you do them three times a week, so much the better. But if you've never strength-trained, you might want to start with only one or two exercises and work up from there. Also, you don't have to do it all on two or three days. If you want to spread it out, you can do these moves over six days – three of them on one day, the other three the next, then back to the first three. Just don't do the same strength-training exercises two days in a row. As we said earlier, your muscles need a day of rest to recover fully from a proper workout.

THE TARGETED STRENGTH-TRAINING PROGRAMME

The six exercises that form the strength-training portion of the *Strong Women, Strong Hearts* programme were designed to have the greatest impact on the largest number of muscles in the body with as few exercises as possible, so as to streamline the process. While all are good for your cardiovascular system, they confer a lot of other benefits as well, which you'll see as you read on.

EXERCISE 1: DIPS ◆

This exercise strengthens your thigh and hip muscles, making it easier to walk and go up and down stairs and hills. It also improves balance and coordination – even your spatial awareness.

Starting position: Stand with good posture, your body facing the banister of a staircase, your left foot on a stair and your right foot parallel but just to the right and off the stair. Hold gently on to the banister with your hands for balance. If you don't have access to a staircase, use a store-bought step next to a kitchen worktop. The step needs to be only 15cm (6in) high.

1-2-3-Down: Lower yourself by bending your left leg so that your right foot drops down below the stair by about 10–15cm (4–6in). You will need to bend at the waist. Your buttocks will be back and your chest high.

Pause for a breath.

1-2-Up: Bring yourself back up to the starting position.

Reps and sets: Repeat the move 12 times on each side – this is one set. Rest for thirty seconds to a minute and then do a second set.

Focal points: Do not let your leading knee go in front of your toes. You will need to engage your abdominal muscles during the movement to stabilize your body.

Progressions
1. Perfect your form by first holding gently on to the banister or worktop for balance.
2. Once you can perform this safely, do the exercise without holding.
3. When you can perform this exercise safely without holding on to the banister or worktop, hold a 1.5–2.5kg (3–5lb) dumbbell in each hand, keeping your hands down at your sides at hip level. Continue to maintain proper form in your upper body when using dumbbells. This is a very difficult level; many people never reach this point. Only progress to this level if you feel safe and comfortable.

EXERCISE 2: LUNGE ◆

The lunge targets a large amount of muscle mass in the body, strengthening the thigh, back and buttocks. It also improves balance and coordination.

Starting position: Stand next to a chair or worktop with your feet hip-width apart, knees slightly bent. Lightly hold on to the chair.

1-2-3-Forward: Take a large step forward with your right leg. Land on the heel of your right foot, then roll your foot forward until it is flat on the floor. Keeping your body erect, bend both knees so that your hips drop straight down. Your front thigh should be almost parallel to the floor and the knee of your back leg should approach the floor. The knee of your forward leg should be over your ankle, not past your toes.

Pause for a breath.

Return: Push back forcefully with the front leg to return to the starting position.

Reps and sets: Alternate legs as you step forward until you have done 12 reps with each leg – this is one set. Rest for thirty seconds to a minute and do a second set.

Focal Points: Do not use the chair to support your weight by leaning on it. Use it only for balance. Maintain posture in the upper body as you descend and ascend, keeping your shoulders and head in line with your hips. Keep the forward leg over the ankle (not in front of it) and in line with the toes. Depending on how tall you are, you may need to adjust the distance between your feet. Distribute your weight between the balls and heels of your feet and equally between the front and back leg. You'll feel the effort in your thighs and back.

Progressions
1. Use the chair for balance and lower with both knees. If you cannot maintain good form when you rise, decrease the distance of your descent. Increase the intensity as you get stronger by dropping down closer to the floor and increasing the distance between your legs.
2. When you are stronger and have more stability and the intensity level drops below a 4, increase the intensity by not using the chair for balance.
3. When you can perform this exercise without using your hand for balance and the intensity drops below a 4, hold a 1.5–2.5kg (3–5lb) dumbbell in each hand while you do the exercise. Progress to 4kg (8lb), 4.5kg (10lb) and 5.5kg (12lb) as you get stronger. This is a very difficult level; many people never reach this point. Progress to this level only if you feel safe and comfortable.

EXERCISE 3: OVERHEAD PRESS ◆

The overhead press feels more difficult and more uncomfortable for many women than a lot of other strength-training moves – at least at first. This is because the muscles needed to perform the exercise – the triceps in the upper arms and the deltoids in the shoulders – are often fairly weak. In addition, women tend not to have flexibility in their shoulder muscles, which this exercise also targets. But the benefits make this an exercise worth sticking with. Strengthening the triceps and shoulder muscles *and* the upper back muscles allows for better movements over your head, such as placing a heavy suitcase in the overhead luggage compartment.

Starting position: You may do this exercise standing or seated in a chair. Your back should be straight, with your head in line with your spine. Hold the dumbbells with palms facing out, shoulder-width apart or slightly more, at a level with your shoulders. Your thumbs will be pointing towards your neck. The dumbbells will be parallel to the floor. Relax your shoulders down your back.

1-2-Up: Press the weights up over your head in a straight line. Do not lock your elbows. Your arms will be above your head and just slightly in front of the plane of your body.

Pause for one second, relaxing your shoulders.

1-2-3-Down: Lower the weights to the starting position.

Reps and sets: Repeat the move 12 times – this is one set. Rest for about thirty seconds to a minute and then do a second set.

Focal points: Keep your upper trunk still during the movement. Initiate the movement in the shoulders. Do not arch your back. The weight is too heavy if you cannot lift it over your head without arching your back. Visualize your shoulders travelling down as you press up. When holding the weights, keep your wrists neutral with your hands fully closed around the dumbbells. Avoid letting the weights bring your wrists too far back or too far forward.

Progressions
1. Start with a 1.5kg (3lb) weight in each hand.
2. As you become stronger and the intensity level decreases below a 4, increase the weight of the dumbbells by 500g–1.5kg (1–3lb) increments per workout to reach a 4 on the intensity scale.

Modifications: If you have any shoulder or elbow pain, try rotating your palms towards your neck for the starting position and maintain this position throughout the lift. Also try keeping your hands shoulder-width apart and no farther.

EXERCISE 4: BICEPS CURL ◆

The biceps are the muscles in the front of your upper arm and they get a lot of use, as you'll see when you strengthen them. A basket of laundry, a child, a bag of groceries – they'll all be easier to lift as your biceps get stronger. Do not be concerned that you will end up with huge bicep bulges. This exercise, like all other strength-training moves, firms and tones you and makes you feel more confident about wearing a sleeveless blouse. It will not make you muscle-bound.

Starting position: Stand with good posture, your feet shoulder-width apart, arms at your sides and your palms facing your thighs, a dumbbell in each hand.

1-2-Up: Slowly rotate your forearms and lift the weights as you bring the dumbbells towards your shoulders. Keep your arms and elbows close to your sides – as if you had a newspaper tucked under each arm. Your palms should be facing your shoulders at the end but not touching them.

Pause for a breath.

1-2-3-Down: Slowly lower your arms to the starting position.

Reps and sets: Repeat the move 12 times – this is one set. Rest for thirty seconds to a minute and then do a second set.

Focal points: Don't let your upper arms or elbows move away from the sides of your body and keep your wrists straight throughout the move. Hold the dumbbells securely, but don't clench your fists around them.

Progressions

1. Start with a 1.5kg (3lb) weight in each hand.
2. As you become stronger and the intensity level decreases below a 4, increase the weight of the dumbbells by 500g–1.5kg (1–3lb) increments per workout to reach a 4 on the intensity scale.

EXERCISE 5: BACK EXTENSION ◆

This exercise strengthens the muscles in your back and buttocks, relieving stress you may feel in your lumbar region or lower back. It will make activities such as raking leaves, shovelling snow and vacuuming easier.

Starting position: Lie facedown with your forehead resting on the floor, legs stretched back, toes pointing back. Extend your left arm straight overhead so that it aligns with your body. Keep your other arm at your side. Tuck your tailbone under you slightly (same as pushing your pubic bone into the floor).

1-2-Up: As you inhale, slowly lift your left arm and right leg off the ground. Keep your arm and leg at the same level. As you lift your arm, your upper back, head and neck will rise, too. Keep your head, neck and back in alignment.

Hold the position for three to five seconds.

1-2-3-Down: Exhale as you lower back to the ground.

Sets and reps: Repeat the move 12 times on each side – this is one set. Rest for thirty seconds to a minute and then do a second set.

Focal points: Think of extending up rather than crunching through the lower back. Keep your shoulders back and your chest broadening as you rise and lower down. Keep your head in alignment with your arm; don't overarch your head and neck up. Feel the move throughout your entire back and down into your upper thighs.

EXERCISE 6: ABDOMINAL CURL ◆

Abdominal curls are the *yang* to the back extension's *ying*. They make your abs tighter and complement your stronger back muscles, thus improving overall posture. Incidentally, strengthening the abdominal muscles literally tucks in your tummy – *without* the discomfort of a girdle.

Starting position: Lie faceup, bending your knees but keeping your feet flat on the floor. Make sure your heels are 30–60cm (1–2ft) from your backside. Interlock your fingers behind the back of your head. This will help to support both your head and your neck as you go through the motion.

1-2-Up: Lift your head and shoulders off the ground by *slowly* contracting your abdominal muscles. You need to bring your back only 8–13cm (3 5in) off the floor. Your chin should be in the neutral position, slightly tucked in but not touching your chest.

Pause for a breath.

1-2-3-Down: Slowly return to the starting position.

Reps and sets: Repeat the move 12 times – this is one set. Rest for thirty seconds to a minute and then do a second set.

Focal Points: When you raise your head, don't pull down with your hands. And don't keep it bent too far forward towards your chest. If your fist fits comfortably between your chin and upper chest, you're doing it right. Also, check for tension – and relax. Think of your stomach as a sponge that is being squeezed. This will help you isolate the right muscles.

THE FLEXIBILITY COMPONENT

The goal of aerobic exercise is to push the heart and the rest of the cardio-vascular system. The goal of strength training is to work the muscles in order for them to adapt and get stronger and also to be more metabolically active. The goal of flexibility is to stretch your muscles, tendons and ligaments so they become more supple and resistant to injury. You need to exceed your current range of motion for the body to respond and increase that range.

While you'll feel the effects of strength training within two weeks, flexibility comes with time; gains are made in 0.5–1cm (¼–½in) increments. But they'll eventually lead to greater freedom of movement, not to mention fewer aches and pains and a reduced risk of injury.

Before You Begin

Never stretch without being warmed up. You don't want to 'snap' your 'rubber bands' before you've 'loosened' them. But that shouldn't be a problem because you'll be doing your stretching at the end of aerobic and strength-training workouts. (Women who start to do even more athletic training – training for running races or competing in triathlons – need to stretch *before* exercising, too, to minimize overuse injuries.)

Note that a stretch may produce some discomfort, at least at first, but it should never be painful. Use common sense. If your muscle quivers or if pain persists, you've stretched too much.

Perform each stretch twice. The movements should be slow and deliberate – and then static (not bouncing) for a period of time when you reach your stretching endpoint (the point at which you feel tight but not in pain).

Try to stretch for at least twenty seconds. That's the *minimum* amount you'll need to see gain. Stretching for thirty seconds to a minute is *optimal.*

It's a good idea to stretch every single day – even on those days you do no other exercises. The greatest increases in flexibility come with stretching every day.

HAMSTRING STRETCH ◆

Stand with your feet hip-width apart, knees slightly bent. Do not lock your knees. Pull your tailbone underneath you slightly. Bend forward from the hips and place your outstretched hands on a chair (or a table if the chair is too low). Keep your neck in line with your spine. Centre your hips over your ankles. You will feel a stronger stretch in the back of the thighs when you do this. Only bend down as far as you can while maintaining a straight back. You will benefit more by doing this stretch properly but not going down as far and you will avoid injuring your back. Complete the stretch twice for twenty seconds. When you are ready, increase the time to thirty seconds or more.

CROSSOVER FOR BUTTOCKS AND HIPS ◆

Lie on your back on the floor with your legs extended. Stretch your left arm out in line with your shoulder. Grasp the outside of your left knee or thigh with your right hand. Inhale and, as you exhale, pull your left knee across your body towards the floor. Keep your shoulders and head on the floor. Pull your left leg across your body until you feel the stretch in the outside of your left hip. You may also feel it on the left side of your trunk. Do the same stretch on your right side for the right hip and buttock. Complete the stretch twice for twenty seconds on both sides. When you are ready, increase the time to thirty seconds or more.

QUADRICEPS STRETCH ◆

Stand behind a chair. Bend your left knee, bring your heel towards your
buttocks and grasp your foot with your left hand. Pull your heel towards
your buttocks. Do not arch your lower back to get your heel closer. Keep
your knee in line with your hip; do not pull it out, in, forward or back.
Keep the knee of your right leg bent slightly throughout the move to avoid
straining it. Complete the stretch twice for twenty seconds on both sides.
When you are ready, increase the time to thirty seconds or more. If you are
unable to grasp your foot because you are not yet flexible enough, place
your lower leg on a second chair behind you.

SHOULDER STRETCH ◆

Stand with your feet hip-width apart, knees slightly bent. Relax your shoulders down and back and keep your head in line with your spine. Interlock your fingers, turn your palms out and stretch your arms forward. (If you can't turn your wrists enough to interlock your fingers, bend your wrists back as far as they will go and touch the fingertips of your two hands together.) Lift them up towards your head, keeping your shoulders down and back. Keep raising your arms until you feel a stretch in your shoulders.

As you lift, do not arch your lower back or drop your head forward. Relax
and breathe throughout the stretch. The maximum endpoint is with your
arms straight above your shoulders, elbows next to your ears. Keep turning
your palms away from you. You will also feel this stretch in the forearms. It
does not matter how far you raise your arms, just that the posture is correct
and you feel a stretch. Complete the stretch twice, twenty seconds each
time. When you are ready, increase the time to thirty seconds or more.

KEEPING TRACK

The best way to ensure that you do the appropriate amount of exercise is to keep a log. Research has shown over and over again that people who keep records of the exercises they do (and the meals and snacks they eat) are the ones most likely to stick to their plan. It forces you to be accountable to yourself. Write in your log and it 'talks back' to you, letting you see where you've kept up and where you've lapsed and need to redouble your efforts.

You can use Miriam's *Strong Women's Journal* or the exercise log below. Simply make multiple copies and keep them in a folder.

GENERAL ACTIVITY Sports games, leisure play, commuting, errands, climbing the stairs, work around the house or garden Goal: as often as you can		
DAY	ACTIVITY	TIME
PLANNED AEROBIC ACTIVITY Goal: 3 to 6 times per week, 30 minutes or more per session		
DAY	ACTIVITY	TIME

STRENGTH TRAINING Goal: 2 to 3 times per week			
EXERCISE 2 SETS/12 REPS	DAY: POUNDS OR '√'	DAY: POUNDS OR '√'	DAY: POUNDS OR '√'
Dips			
Lunges			
Biceps Curl			
Overhead Press			
Abdominal Curl			
Back Extension			
FLEXIBILITY Goal: After each exercise session			
STRETCHES	'√'	'√'	'√'
Hamstring			
Crossover			
Quadriceps			
Shoulders			

STEPS PER DAY (IF YOU USE A PEDOMETER)

Monday	Tuesday	Wednesday	Thursday	Friday	Saturday	Sunday
___	___	___	___	___	___	___

WHAT'S NEXT?

While there's nothing like an exercise routine to ground you, the repetitiveness can become 'stale' after a while, which can make the programme difficult to stick to.

Feel free to vary the types of exercises you do. Even if you keep doing the same activities, such as brisk walking, some people enjoy finding new places to walk. The visual stimulation of looking at new things could be enough to keep you going. Or you could cross-train: walk one day, swim another and bike another.

When it comes to strength training, the exercises here certainly cover the gamut of what your body needs but they are by no means the only ones. We encourage you to vary your strength-training programme. Check out one of Miriam's other books; join a fitness centre where you can work out on machines; hire a personal trainer for a few sessions to freshen up your routine. You can also learn several different exercise routines by going to www.strongwomen.com or getting some help at a health club. Even if you don't belong to a gym, many of them let you buy a day pass and you can get strength-training tips from certified trainers on staff.

Helen knows well the value of varying your routine. Along with using a treadmill at the YWCA (plus resistance machines), she enjoys hiking, bicycling and, during the winter, cross-country skiing. She actually *looks forward* to exercising. 'I don't even think about the fact that I'm protecting my heart as I go,' she says. 'I just like what I'm doing and I love how I feel when I finish a session.'

CHAPTER 7

Ten Tough Strategies for Weight Loss – That Work!

I had been overweight my entire life, even as a child. The only time I wasn't overweight was when I was born. Four years ago, I decided it was time to take charge of my health. I was over 19 stone and a size 26. My blood cholesterol was undeniably high – 227; my blood pressure, in the hypertensive range – 140/82. Also contributing to my decision: the horrifying experience of having to get off a ride at an amusement park because the safety bar wouldn't lock over me.

I knew I needed a two-pronged approach: I had to eat properly and I had to exercise.

I really had to change the way I ate. If you look at my dinner plate now, it's going to be two helpings of vegetables and maybe a potato and some type of protein. Before, it was a huge piece of meat, a huge baked potato and a small helping of one type of vegetable.

Also, fruit has become my major snack now. Once in a while I have a fat-free pudding or popcorn with just a little bit of butter. Before, it was a biscuit or cake or a sweet.

As far as exercise, I started out slowly, but I kept at it.

Nine months into the whole thing, I had lost over 4 stone and joined a gym. Two years after I started, I had lost nearly 9 stone. I now weigh 10 stone and wear a size 12. I have maintained this weight for two and a half years. My cholesterol is 169; my blood pressure, 118/76 – normal. Not only have I improved my heart health, I have also lost my migraine headaches, my stomach problems, my foot aches and my backaches. I cannot even begin to describe the feeling of being healthy after all those years.

– DEANNE

Two-thirds of all women in the US are either overweight or obese; and over a half in the UK. That raises the risk for heart disease sevenfold. Weight management is critical. But as with other lifestyle changes, there's no one right way to do it. Deanne, for instance, says she was 'a junk-food junkie' and had to initiate changes by substituting more healthy, lower-calorie foods for less nutritious, high-calorie choices. She also says she had to teach herself about portion sizes, remarking that 'it was nothing to eat half a box of pasta' before she began to lose weight. Furthermore, she had to begin asking herself many times throughout the day, 'Am I really hungry?' If the answer was no, she'd take a few minutes to walk away from the food she wanted to let the wave, or craving, pass. In other words, she made the effort her own, separating her larger goal into various smaller components that she could keep chipping away at.

Her strategy couldn't have been better. For weight loss, breaking down the goal into simple rules that you can keep track of as you go along makes it much easier. After all, you can't wake up one day and somehow be thinner 'cold turkey', the way you can give up cigarettes.

That's where this chapter comes in. We have identified the ten most important guidelines for weight loss – the ones that really make a difference if followed by women who want to finally reach their goal of losing weight to become healthier. That said, however, these guidelines, while tough, are flexible enough that they can be adapted to any lifestyle. They will also help women who are currently at a healthy weight *maintain* that weight as they get older.

Unfortunately, women who are currently at a healthy weight are in the minority. As we said before, more than half of all women in the UK are either overweight or out-and-out obese. And the extra weight is substantially increasing their risk for heart disease, so for the sake of their health, it's important that they try to take off some of it. By the same token, many who are not overweight have to work hard to keep creeping pounds at bay. Especially after major life changes, such as getting married, having a baby, getting a divorce, losing a spouse or after menopause, pounds have a sneaky way of showing up – and raising blood cholesterol, blood pressure and blood sugar, which in turn raise heart disease risk.

It is by no means necessary to be stick thin to get your risk for heart disease as low as possible. For instance, a woman who is 5ft 4in tall and weighs 10 stone 4lb is at a healthy weight. Furthermore, in many women who weigh substantially more than is good for them, losing even just 10 or 20 pounds is enough to significantly reduce blood pressure, blood cholesterol and blood sugar levels – sometimes to the point that women taking medication no longer need it, or can at least have their dose reduced.

What Do You Have to Lose?

How overweight are you? Twenty pounds? Fifty pounds? More? How did you decide? A lot of women go by the weight they were in high school, or the weight they'd need to be to fit into a certain size. We are constantly amazed when we talk to women about the 'creative' ways in which they come up with the amount of weight they need to lose. For instance: 'When I was twenty-one, I weighed 8 stone 3lb. Now I'm fifty-seven, have gone through menopause and have had three children, but that is really the weight that worked for me. Yes, I know I weigh 12 stone 12lb now, but that is where I want to be.'

That's not realistic. Healthy weight is not a wish; it is a scientific number. Actually, there is more than just the number on the scale that says whether you're at a healthy weight. A number that scientists often use is called your body mass index, or BMI, which is a given weight for a given height.

In the scientific community, a healthy BMI is anything between 19 and 24. Overweight is a BMI of 25 through 29 and obese is 30 or more. What is *your* BMI? To find out, you need to measure your height and get an accurate body weight.

Measure those two numbers in the morning with no clothes or shoes on. Then look for your height at the left side of the table. Go across the column until you get to the number you weigh on the scale and look at the top of the column to see what BMI your weight corresponds to.

Body Mass Index

1. Read down the first column to locate your height in inches.
2. Read across that row and locate your weight in pounds.
3. Read the heading on top of the column – that's your BMI.

UNDERWEIGHT BMI under 19		HEALTHY WEIGHT BMI 19–25							OVERWEIGHT BMI 26–29			
HEIGHT (inches)	18 or less	19	20	21	22	23	24	25	26	27	28	29
58	86	91	96	100	105	110	115	119	124	129	134	138
59	89	94	99	104	109	114	119	124	128	133	138	143
60	92	97	102	107	112	118	123	128	133	138	143	148
61	95	100	106	111	116	122	127	132	137	143	148	153
62	98	104	109	115	120	126	131	136	142	147	153	158
63	101	107	113	118	124	130	135	141	146	152	158	163
64	105	110	116	122	128	134	140	145	151	157	163	169
65	108	114	120	126	132	138	144	150	156	162	168	174
66	111	118	124	130	136	142	148	155	161	167	173	179
67	115	121	127	134	140	146	153	159	166	172	178	185
68	118	125	131	138	144	151	158	164	171	177	184	190
69	122	128	135	142	149	155	162	169	176	182	189	196
70	125	132	139	146	153	160	167	174	181	188	195	202
71	129	136	143	150	157	165	172	179	186	193	200	208
72	132	140	147	154	162	169	177	184	191	199	206	213

Very Overweight BMI 30–39										Extremely Overweight
30	31	32	33	34	35	36	37	38	39	40 or more
143	148	153	158	162	167	172	177	181	186	191+
148	153	158	163	168	173	178	183	188	193	198+
153	158	163	168	174	179	184	189	194	199	204+
158	164	169	174	180	185	190	195	201	206	211+
164	169	175	180	186	191	196	202	207	213	218+
169	175	180	186	191	197	203	208	214	220	225+
174	180	186	192	197	204	209	215	221	227	232+
180	186	192	198	204	210	216	222	228	234	240+
186	192	198	204	210	216	223	229	235	241	247+
191	198	204	211	217	223	230	236	242	249	255+
197	203	210	216	223	230	236	243	249	256	262+
203	209	216	223	230	236	243	250	257	263	270+
209	216	223	229	236	243	250	257	264	271	278+
215	222	229	236	243	250	257	265	272	279	286+
221	228	235	242	250	258	265	272	279	287	294+

We suggest you set small goals – one unit of BMI at a time, which is the equivalent of about 5 pounds (unless you're on the tall side, in which case a single BMI unit can be 6 or 7 pounds). If you're obese, reducing by one BMI unit at a time will slowly but surely get you into the overweight zone. If you're overweight, it will move you slowly towards healthy weight.

For those women who *are* at a healthy weight but have high cholesterol or high blood pressure because over the years they have gone from a BMI of 22 to a BMI of 24, dropping down one or two BMI units will likely lower their risk factors.

Try not to focus simply on weight and BMI by themselves. Focus instead on the *behaviours* we delineate in this chapter, which will help you get to your goal weight.

Of course, as many of you know firsthand, losing weight and keeping it off over the long term is not that easy, helpful guidelines notwithstanding. And, unlike so many diet books that promise you'll never go hungry if you just eat low-carbohydrate or high-protein foods or follow some other gimmick, we are not going to pretend that it is. Because the truth of the matter is that you probably *will* experience some hunger or feelings of deprivation, at least at first, since **the only way you can make real headway in a weight-loss effort is to eat fewer calories than you are used to.** It's perhaps the most difficult health behaviour task you'll ever need to engage in. A colleague of ours who had to lose some weight to bring down her blood cholesterol says the first few days in particular were rough, in part because she felt hungry and in part because she was having to re-evaluate the way she had always approached food.

THE TEN STRATEGIES FOR EFFECTIVE WEIGHT LOSS

The following ten strategies really *will* make the going a little easier. There are no tricks here, but there *is* a certain alchemy that can be achieved by bringing all the elements of these guidelines together in one effort. That is, while the guidelines are simple on the face of it, their sum is very powerful. Incorporate them into your lifestyle and you will find it hard *not* to lose excess weight.

Indeed, many of them are put to use by people enrolled in the US National Weight Loss Registry. To join this registry, which is maintained by researchers at Brown University and now includes thousands of names, a person has to have lost at least 30 pounds and have kept off the weight for at least one year. But the average registrant has lost about *60* pounds and maintained the loss for roughly *five* years!

The ten strategies are divided along two general lines. There are rules about your eating *behaviours* and *mind-set and* rules related specifically to the *foods* you eat and the *calories* you expend in physical activity.

1. Believe You Can Lose Weight and Commit to Making the Necessary Changes in Your Diet.

Sounds like fluff, right? Believe you can lose the weight and you will. Well, the evidence shows that you really do have to turn on a 'belief' switch in your head. In the mid-1990s, researchers at the University of Maryland tracked more than fifty women who were following a diet and exercise programme for almost a year. Before the programme began, the women were asked whether they thought they'd lose weight. A little more than half – the believers – said yes. The rest expected to fail. Nine months later, those who had trusted in their ability to lose weight at the beginning lost 30 per cent more weight than those who didn't have much hope for themselves.

Why is believing in yourself so crucial? It helps strengthen your commitment to a task that's going to take a considerable amount of mental and emotional energy, a task that may very well go two steps forwards, one step back. After all, you're going to veer from your plan *sometimes and* it's at those times most of all that you need to have faith in yourself to be able to get right back on track rather than tell yourself you're a failure who can't stick to anything. That way, a candy bar, for instance, remains what it is – a single candy bar rather than 'proof' that you have no willpower. Another way of putting it: having faith in your ability to commit to lifestyle changes that will lead to weight loss will help you stay with it for the long haul. Deanne knows this firsthand. 'There were many times that I would slip,' she says. 'But I made sure I bounced right back and didn't beat myself up about it.'

2. Write Down Every Single Thing You Eat.

Consider the research. In one weight-loss study conducted in California, researchers asked half the participants to write down everything they ate.

There was no counseling on *what* foods to eat, *how much* to eat, *when* to eat, etc. The upshot: those who kept food diaries lost more weight. In another study, investigators found that the best predictor for shedding pounds was not exercise intensity or body weight or anything else that typically goes with dieting. It was whether or not people kept a food journal.

What is it about writing down all the foods (and beverages) they eat that helps people stick to their diets? One thing is that it makes it harder to rationalize going overboard. Once you put the foods you eat 'outside of yourself' and onto the page, you can't convince yourself that you 'really didn't eat that much'. It's all there, right in front of you – whether you took seconds, nibbled on something in the car and so on.

But perhaps even more important, writing down your foods keeps the weight-loss effort front and centre at all times. You can't just eat and forget about it. You have to *count up* your food choices.

Writing it down also increases commitment and motivation. There's nothing like seeing something in black and white to keep from veering off track. At the same time, seeing that you've made good food choices ratchets up resolve – you're less inclined to mess up the hard work you've already done.

To get the most out of this, *always jot down when you eat as well as under what circumstances. You'll pick up eating patterns you may never have realized.* For instance, perhaps you'll discover that you tend to overeat just before or after late-afternoon work meetings. Maybe you'll find you eat much more than you thought while standing in the kitchen after clearing the dinner dishes. Once you begin to pick up your patterns, you can begin to work through solutions for *breaking* them. It could be as simple as reminding yourself that once you leave the table, dinner is over and that a couple of bites here and there could add up to 100 calories (10 pounds in a year's time).

We are so convinced of the value of writing down all the foods you eat that Miriam's book, *The Strong Women's Journal,* makes it easy to record every single day's food choices.

3. Commit to Breakfast.

Both of us are big believers in breakfast. As we previously illustrated, it's a meal at which it's easy to get things lacking in the western diet: calcium (from low- or non-fat yogurt, milk or cheese); fruit (on top of cereal or mixed into yogurt); and whole grains (in the cereal itself or a slice of whole-wheat toast). Also, if you start the day off with a nutritious breakfast, you'll be less inclined to play fast and loose with your weight-loss effort later in the day. People tend to build on their positive acts. One step towards weight control leads to the next.

But now there's another reason to make sure to eat breakfast as part of a weight-loss plan. Research out of the University of Texas in the US analyzed seven days' worth of diet diaries kept by almost 900 women and men and found that eating a hearty meal earlier in the day proved more satiating than the same number of calories eaten later on and thereby blunted overall calorie consumption. In other words, eating a substantial breakfast may work *biologically* to keep you from eating less after nightfall.

The numbers are not hard and fast and are going to be different for different people, but the gist is as follows. Say you consume only 150 calories at breakfast – a slice of toast with margarine and a cup of coffee with milk. You might end up totalling 2,000 calories for the entire day. But if you eat 300 to 400 calories at breakfast – maybe a serving of wholegrain cereal with fresh or frozen berries and a banana with a cup of skimmed milk, along with coffee – you might eat only 1,800 calories by the time the day is over.

Why do people seem to feel more sated by food eaten earlier in the day? The biological mechanism hasn't been worked out, but it could be that the body is set to certain diurnal rhythms that don't agree with the current human lifestyle. That is, maybe our mechanism for feeling full is in full swing in the morning, when we need enough calories to get through the day. But then it shuts off when the sun goes down because throughout most of our evolutionary history, people pretty much went to sleep at nightfall and therefore didn't need to feel sated to conduct more activity.

Of course, today, with artificial light created by electricity, people remain active long into the evening, with lots of opportunities to eat and not feel sated. Indeed, in the University of Texas research, as the day wore on, the intervals between eating episodes lessened – regardless of the number of calories eaten. Think of it in terms of your own lifestyle. It might be hours between breakfast and lunch but a relatively short time between a rather heavy dinner and a high-calorie snack between dinner and bedtime.

We don't want to suggest that eating too little at breakfast is the only reason people overeat at night. It's not. There's television watching, boredom, eating to de-stress and all sorts of other reasons. But since eating a reasonably substantial breakfast can potentially curb the trend and provide a healthy first meal at the same time, along with motivating you to keep on track as you start your day, we wholeheartedly support it.

Breakfast doesn't have to be eaten soon after you wake up. Some people, Alice included, often aren't hungry as soon as they awake and take their breakfast to work with them. Delaying breakfast is okay – as long as it happens!

4. Eat Only at a Table Designated for Dining – Whether It's in Your Kitchen, Dining Room or Office – *without the TV.*

Thirty years ago, you would never have seen someone eating a doughnut on a bus, or wolfing down a slice of pizza while walking along the street or chomping on take-away fare in the car. Meals were eaten around a table – without the television on. But with the explosion of cheap, highly palatable convenience foods, people's whole way of eating has changed. And we believe it has contributed to the precipitous rise in body weight seen in recent decades.

When you eat on the run, you tend to eat extremely fast – too fast for your brain to pick up signals of satiety from your stomach. It takes about twenty minutes for the GI tract to inform the brain that you're full. If you're eating really fast because you want to finish a 500-calorie burger or pastry before you reach the sliproad to a dual carriageway, or because you're trying to do twenty things at once and aren't focusing on your food, or because you're in the family room watching TV and not paying attention, you can end up consuming a lot more calories than your body is actually hungry for. If you sit at a table, on the other hand, you're eating *mindfully.* You're focusing on the food, which in itself slows things down.

You're also tasting your food better – slower chewing allows for a fuller gustatory experience, with more flavours and textures perceived. That, too, can cut down on the amount you eat because you feel more satisfied with less.

Eating in a relaxed manner has the same effect. The more you enjoy the dining *experience,* the less you need to get what you need out of it by heaping on more food. And the less you'll hurriedly sneak in a lot of calories without realizing it, say, by tasting too often while cooking, finishing the leftovers in the serving dish or eating what a small child has left on her or his plate. All of these things tend *not* to happen in calm moments at the table but in those almost imperceptible, stress-filled moments between not wanting to overdo and having overdone it before you have had a chance to reason with yourself.

We cannot emphasize enough how important it is to make sure you eat all meals and snacks in a relaxed manner without a lot of distractions – including the television. There is a very strong relationship between the amount of TV someone watches and the degree to which she is overweight.

As busy as we both are, we make a point of dining this way. No one ever eats away from the table in either of our houses except for those rare times when someone is sick in bed and is served soup upstairs or, for instance, the family is making a special night of it by watching the Super Bowl and enjoying some popcorn in front of the television. Also, we try hard to leave work every night before six o'clock no matter how busy we are because we want to get home and have dinner with our families.

Those times when meals become haphazard, you are setting yourself up to fail. The eating gets less healthy, the calories are piled on willy-nilly because it's hard to keep track when you're scoffing down foods on the go and all enjoyment of food – which is even more important when you're trying to eat less of it – goes out the window.

Granted, sitting down to meals is not always easy for a family to negotiate. A teenager has swimming practice after school, for instance, or somebody comes home late from work several times a week. But the more you can create a pattern for eating together when it *is* possible, the better attention to calories you are going to be able to pay.

5. Set a Kitchen-Closed Time – and Stick to It.

In a study in Sweden, investigators found that obese women tended to eat the same number of calories as healthy weight women throughout most of the day, yet ate significantly more calories from eight in the evening until midnight.

Perhaps you recognize yourself as an evening eater. A lot of people are and for a lot of reasons – boredom, TV food ads and the list goes on. If you make a pact with yourself not to eat after dinner, you will save hundreds of calories a day. Evening is prime time for ice cream, chocolate, crisps and nuts, all of which can be gobbled in minutes.

People's kitchen-closed times will vary. Some people don't get home from work until late. That is okay. The point is to stop dinner from becoming the beginning of an eating activity that continues until you go to bed.

6. Be Extra Vigilant When You Haven't Prepared the Food Yourself.

Both of us believe firmly that preparing your own meals as often as possible is one of the best ways to limit calories and improve your diet. When you cook the meal, you control what and how much, you're eating. But the reality is that many women are already at their limit time-wise and simply have to rely, at least in part, on restaurant food, take-away food and prepared supermarket foods. Indeed, more than half of all Americans eat at least one meal away from home on any given day, according to a US government survey known as 'What We Eat in America'.

That's why it's so important to be aware that food prepared outside your own kitchen tends to be higher in calories than food you make yourself and that it's important to eat such food with special attention to portion size. A study conducted by some of our colleagues at Tufts makes the point all too well. The researchers looked at the frequency with which thirty-six women and men visited seven different kinds of restaurants, including those that specialized in fried chicken, burgers, pizza, Chinese or Mexican foods and fried fish. The more often the subjects ate out, the higher their calorie consumption and the higher their level of body fatness. It was that simple.

So when you eat out or order in, choose wisely. In a sit-down restaurant, really do ask for at least half the portion to be wrapped up before it's even brought to the table. Or, upon getting something home, immediately put at least half in the fridge for another meal. Don't trust your willpower, which will be in short supply when you're hungry and tired.

And don't be afraid to ask for meals in restaurants exactly as you want them. After all, you're paying for them!

Miriam was in a restaurant in Bellingham, Washington, recently and the waiter was kind enough to reassure her that if she wanted to double the vegetable and halve the potato, that was fine. You really *can* have it your way, even if the restaurant doesn't have a little slogan to prove it.

Alice knows this from experience, too. When she was staying in a New Hampshire inn recently for a little cross-country ski break, she asked for the kitchen to leave out the sauce on her fish, double the vegetables and leave off the scalloped potatoes (which contained cream and butter she didn't want). She was not perceived as difficult. The staff was happy to oblige. If enough of us ask for these types of changes to menus, food will start to be served this way routinely and we won't have to ask anymore.

7. Don't Drink Your Calories.

The calories you drink don't end up making you feel as full as the calories you eat. Researchers at Purdue University in Indiana, USA, made the point when they gave people either 400 calories' worth of sugary jelly beans or 400 calories' worth of sugary soda pop. The people given the jelly beans ate fewer calories later in the day to compensate for their jelly bean consumption. The soda drinkers did not.

Researchers suspect that liquids just don't trigger satiety mechanisms in the gastrointestinal tract in the same way that solids do. Whatever the reason, all the calories Americans now consume from beverages are no doubt contributing to the national epidemic of overweight and obesity. Soft drinks are *the* leading source of added sugars in our diets; consumption of carbonated beverages has risen 500 per cent since the 1950s! Consumption of many kinds of fruit and fruit-based juices and drinks, none of which has any of the fibre of actual fruit, has increased 280 per cent. (And 100 per cent fruit juice tends to have as many calories as sweetened juice beverages. Don't be fooled into thinking that juice per se is relatively low in calories.)

Then there are all the newfangled drinks at coffee shops, many of which have more calories than the pastry or doughnuts sold alongside them. A caramel cappuccino has 350 calories; a white chocolate mocha 440.

We believe every calorie you take in should be *felt*, especially when you're trying to make each calorie count because you're cutting back. And since liquid calories are not well perceived by the body, we feel strongly that thirst should be quenched only by water or a cup of non-fat or 1% milk here or there. If diet soft drinks or coffee or tea sweetened with artificial sweetener help you limit calories, use them. We don't *advocate* use of artificial sweeteners. But for some people, they *can* have a place in a reduced-calorie diet.

8. Eat Grains, But Make Them *Whole* Grains.

As pointed out in chapter 5, some people think that carbohydrates have a special tendency to add fat to the body. They don't. In fact, wholegrain carbohydrates can aid a weight-loss effort. In research conducted here at Tufts, one of our colleagues switched people from refined grains to whole grains, with the result that they started complaining immediately that they were being given too much to eat! They were not getting any more calories. But whole grains, unlike refined, contain fibre, which can help fill you up.

The average person eats only one serving of whole grains per day and six to twelve – or more – servings of refined grains. That many servings even of whole grains is too much, certainly for a weight-loss effort. So our advice here is twofold and while it's simple to say, it takes some planning.

First, while you are actively losing weight, stick only with whole grains. Second, limit whole grains to no more than four to six servings a day. Remember, a serving is a 25g slice of bread, 85g of brown rice or wholewheat pasta, or a portion of wholegrain cereal (oatmeal is a whole grain), as listed on the side of the cereal box. (It's okay to eat 175g of wholewheat pasta at once. Just be sure to count it as two servings.)

Eating only whole grains may be more difficult than you think – at first. Only 5 per cent of the grain-based foods in the supermarket are whole – and probably less in restaurants. But it will really fuel your weight-loss effort, in no small part because it removes from your eating plan a lot of foods people tend to overdo: ordinary pasta, cakes and biscuits (both made with white flour), oversized bagels (a 150g bagel is the caloric equivalent of five slices of white bread), pretzels and most crackers.

9. Snack Smart.

We wholeheartedly endorse snacking, as our menus show. It staves off hunger between meals and provides an opportunity to consume essential nutrients.

But a snack is not a 200-calorie energy or candy bar or a 150-calorie bag of crisps. It's an 80-calorie apple or a 120-calorie cup of non-fat yogurt.

How do you get yourself to eat those foods instead of biscuits, candy bars and so on? Buy them and not the other stuff – and keep them front and centre either in a fruit bowl on the kitchen worktop or right in front of the refrigerator on an eye-level shelf; or in your handbag at work so they are readily available. *You* control the snack choices.

Interestingly, there has been some research associating low- and non-fat dairy foods like yogurt with weight control. Two recent studies have found that in both women and men, a diet rich in low-fat dairy products was linked with lower body weight. Other preliminary research has found, similarly, that increased servings of dairy products are associated with lower body *fat*.

Why isn't clear. Most likely, dairy products are a marker for eating healthily in general. Another speculation is that dairy products may stimulate weight loss by increasing fat metabolism. The effect, if there indeed is one, is modest. We are not at all pretending that if you just add dairy foods to your diet, you'll magically lose a lot of extra weight. But since two to three servings of dairy foods are needed each day for general good health anyway, snacks are a good place to incorporate them. Just be sure they're low in fat – and sugar. A lot of yogurts are loaded with sugar, which can increase calories considerably.

Also, *plan ahead*. Make sure to always have fresh fruit and dairy at home or bring it to the office. When the 4.30 afternoon lull hits, you want to have the right snack on hand.

10. Move Your Body.

It's not impossible to lose weight without exercise, but it's certainly difficult – and not good for you, either. Almost every single person in the US National Weight Control Registry exercises regularly, by which we mean almost every day. They know intuitively what a American National Institutes of Health Task Force on Obesity stated several years ago. When you're trying to lose weight, 75 per cent of the calorie deficit comes from eating less food – and 25 per cent comes from burning more calories through increased physical activity. The weight-loss registrants have also learned what studies keep showing: nine in ten weight losers who do not exercise gain the weight back.

Walking is the most convenient form of exercise. A 10 stone 10lb woman will burn 80 to 100 calories for each mile she walks. Of course, even walking just one mile might seem daunting to someone who needs to lose a substantial amount of weight but hasn't exercised in years – or perhaps ever. Likewise, as we discussed in chapter 6, lifting weights to rev up metabolism could also be difficult for someone who has never strength-trained.

Don't take our word for it; take Deanne's. Exercising 'wasn't easy,' she comments. 'I remember the early days of lifting cans of baked beans and one-litre bottles of water. I soon progressed to 2.5kg (5lb) and 4.5kg (10lb) weights and more and more walking on the treadmill. A year and a half after starting, I even discovered that I liked running. I had tried many times over the years to run but always hated it. I guess I finally hit a weight at which it became enjoyable.'

SLOW AND STEADY WINS THE RACE

You may not want to tackle all ten of our strategies all at once. That's okay. But if you are going to make a serious attempt at losing weight, you are going to need to tackle most of them or else find your own healthy way to lose the pounds. In the end you need to eat less and move more. Right now, think about which strategies you are going to adopt first and how you are going to do so.

We have found with many women that each step is a building block that propels them on to others. Start small, as Deanne did and before long you'll have an arsenal of weight-loss approaches that you're employing to make the most of your weight-loss efforts as quickly as possible.

But do start. If you are overweight, you simply are not going to shed any excess pounds without making some serious adjustments to your daily habits – that could take getting used to. If you wait until you feel 'just right' about it, you could go your whole life weighing more than you should. There will always be something getting in your way, so you might as well jump in *now* – not tomorrow morning – and get the ball rolling. Make the switch in your brain to one of commitment and belief. It won't feel as difficult after a week or two of building the changes into your routine.

Says Deanne, 'After a while, losing weight becomes a self-fulfilling thing. The more you lose, the easier it gets to keep it up. In my case, my self-esteem and confidence were soaring as my dress size was dropping.

'At some point every day I still have to make a decision not to eat something that's not good for me or that I'm not hungry for. There's no day that goes by where I don't get challenged. But I've learned to listen to my body. I make smarter choices. It really has got easier.'

CHAPTER 8

Relaxing, Taking a Deep Breath and Other Approaches

◆

Your heart 'races' or 'pounds' from stress or anger. 'Skips a beat' when you feel afraid. 'Sinks' when you're low or depressed. Even if you've never made the connection consciously, the fact that our emotions and our hearts are inextricably interwoven is so well intuited that the notion is embedded in our very language.

The Bible itself makes reference to it. When Jacob heard that his son, Joseph, had been alive the entire twenty-two years he had been missing in Egypt, his heart 'fell' from the shock. Biblical scholars have interpreted it to mean that he suffered a heart attack.

Today, a growing body of research is beginning to confirm scientifically what people have always known 'in their hearts': stress, whether experienced as anxiety, depression or some other emotion, affects cardiovascular health. A lot of the evidence centres around the impact of emotional health in heart disease that has already been diagnosed. For instance, it has been shown that depression increases the risk for a second heart attack. But there's more and more evidence that stress, anguish and related mental states play a role in the *development* of heart disease as well.

STRESS AND HOSTILITY'S DIRECT EFFECT

Stress and its influence on the heart can be hard to quantify, but one telling study conducted in Sweden in the 1990s makes the connection. Researchers there compared city bus drivers to bus drivers in rural areas. What they found was that bus drivers in urban situations were more likely to die from heart disease than other workers in the same geographical area, but rural bus drivers had the same rate of heart disease death as other workers in their locale. As anyone who has ever ridden on a city bus knows, driving one entails *a lot* of stress; thus, the researchers concluded, stress played into urban bus drivers' worse rates of cardiovascular death than those experienced by their rural counterparts.

Several studies have also spotlighted anger, including one from the University of North Carolina in the US. Researchers there gave an anger 'test' to some 13,000 people, asking them whether they tended to fly off the handle, say unkind things when angry, or become furious when slowed down by others (think traffic jam or having to re-explain something). The higher they scored, the more likely they were to suffer heart problems down the line. In fact, the most anger-prone people had nearly a threefold greater risk of suffering a heart attack or dying from heart disease than those with a longer fuse.

Another study, conducted at the University of Michigan, showed that hostile people, when asked to relive an angry memory, had larger and longer-lasting rises in blood pressure than others. And a third study, out from California, suggested that hostility starts hurting the heart early in life. Young adults with scores above average on an anger test were more likely than others to have already undergone some calcification in their coronary arteries, which is one of the steps contributing to advanced atherosclerosis.

Along with raising blood pressure and paving the way for the faster development of atherosclerosis, anger is believed to prompt the release of stress hormones such as cortisol and catecholamines. Over the long term, all these stress hormones flooding the system can damage the delicate linings of blood vessels surrounding the heart. They can disrupt the heart's electrical rhythm, too. And they set in motion a process whereby blood platelets become 'stickier' and clump together, which may in turn set the stage for a heart attack or stroke.

Not surprisingly, people with a hostile outlook tend to get themselves into angry confrontations more often, which only sets the whole chain of events into action with a consistency that increases the risk for heart problems that much more.

HOW DEPRESSION TAKES ITS TOLL

Some people have characterized depression as anger turned inward. Whether you subscribe to that definition or not, depression, which affects women disproportionately, can be just as bad for the heart as hostility. Research at Montreal's McGill University has found that depressed people have a three to four times higher risk of dying within eighteen months of having a heart attack.

Another study has found that depressed people are more likely to end up with heart disease in the first place. Ten years after a group of women and men took a depression test at a time when all of them were heart disease-free, those whose test scores showed evidence of depression were 70 per cent more likely than the others to have suffered a heart attack or developed ischemia or some other form of heart disease.

Why? It could be that people with depression have difficulty following lifestyle recommendations to prevent heart problems. Because of their condition, they often cannot take proper care of themselves by adhering to a heart-healthy diet or getting adequate exercise. A Johns Hopkins University School of Medicine study in the USA has shown, in addition, that heart attack survivors diagnosed with depression are less likely than their nondepressed counterparts to adhere to treatment recommendations meant to reduce their risk for a second cardiac event down the line.

But there's more to it than not taking care of themselves. People with depression also have a lower heart rate variability, meaning their hearts are less adaptable to situations and won't change their 'pace' sufficiently when they go, for example, from sitting in a chair to climbing a staircase (refer to the box on page 58).

Furthermore, while depressed people may often seem in low gear, they are actually in a state of high arousal much of the time, just as angry people are. Thus, they release high levels of stress hormones that unduly tax the cardiovascular system. (Depression may look sluggish on the outside but can really be churning up the system from the inside.)

STEPS FOR GAINING EMOTIONAL EQUILIBRIUM

Angry, depressed or just plain stressed out, you don't have to live with the negative state of mind – and let it keep taking a toll on your heart. There's much you can do, literally, to blunt negative emotions, whether that means stopping to smell the roses or seeing the world a little more rose-coloured.

Sometimes it's just a matter of working to see things through a different angle of life's prism. For instance, maybe you have a colleague who always tries to take credit for projects that you have a big hand in bringing forward. Of course it's annoying. But maybe it pays to consider that it might very well make the person look petty to the higher-ups, at least some of whom have to be aware of all your hard work.

Or maybe you often feel stressed because there are frequent delays and interruptions – through no fault of your own – in your already very tightly scheduled day. And those delays make you lose it – you start snapping at your office mates or family. Perhaps the solution is to acknowledge up front that things never run as smoothly as one would like and plan fewer tasks per given amount of time. That may feel like inefficiency, but in the end it could actually be more pragmatic. You get to focus fully on each task at hand and you don't end up angry and disappointed that you weren't able to get more done.

Sometimes even just acknowledging openly to yourself what's gnawing at you can help to put it into proper perspective. It reminds you that there are more dimensions to life than whatever is so troubling at that very moment.

Along with turning life's frustrations on their ear a little, there are a number of anxiety-reducing practices that millions of people use across the globe to get 'centred' and thereby take better care of themselves emotionally – and thereby take better care of their hearts. Check out the ones below to see if any might be right for you.

Meditation (Birkenstocks Not Required)

Many people hear the term 'meditation' and they think it means sitting cross-legged on the floor in flowing robes or a loincloth. It doesn't. In fact, it's a rather mechanical process. For instance, in a type of meditation called *transcendental meditation,* you simply sit for twenty minutes twice a day with your eyes closed. During that quiet time, you repeat a mantra – a soothing sound – that allows the mind and body to settle down, so to speak and 're-lease' stress and hostility. The result is a deep state of restful alertness. That is, the body is at rest, but the mind becomes more wakeful, or lit, from within. That gets the mind and body into balance.

People generally link meditating, or being in a meditative state, with stress reduction. And rightly so. What's less well known is that in some cases, meditation can lower blood pressure as well as drugs can. We believe all types of meditation can have this effect, but the research to date has focused on transcendental meditation, which is why we refer specifically to that type here. In a project involving more than 100 people at California's West Oakland Health Center, those who learned and performed transcendental meditation every day for three months experienced an overall drop in systolic pressure that was greater than the drop in people who simply were counselled on lifestyle changes such as losing excess weight, cutting back on salt and drinking less alcohol. The meditators' diastolic pressure also dropped more than in the group receiving only lifestyle advice. Comparable reductions in blood pressure achieved with drugs have been linked with substantial reductions in stroke risk and congestive heart failure.

Meditation not only lowers blood pressure, but by reducing stress, it can also help people curb unhealthy behaviours that get in the way of their heart-healthy efforts. Consider that people in the Oakland study who did not meditate did not make any appreciable changes in their lifestyle habits. But the meditation group went from roughly eleven drinks a week to five – which, for women, meant going from too much alcohol to an amount that's consistent with protection against heart disease. That, combined with the stress reduction imparted by meditation, could benefit the heart that much more.

For those who want to try meditation, major cities across the country have local centres listed on the website www.t-m.org.uk, or see the Resources section at the back of this book.

Tai Chi

It's now fairly well established that tai chi, an ancient, graceful martial arts form in which slow movements flow one into the other, lowers the body's level

Herbs, Roots and Other Complementary Therapies

Meditation, tai chi, yoga – all of these are effective practices for reducing heart disease risk. But along with *doing* things to ward off heart disease, a lot of women are *taking* substances purported to have heart-helping powers. And those substances are now getting serious scrutiny from the medical community. The US National Institutes of Health is currently devoting considerable resources to studying adjunctive therapies that include plant extracts and other naturally occurring compounds.

To date, the evidence of benefit for many of those substances is slim to non-existent. Until the new research results become available, it is too early to recommend them.

For instance, despite promising results from some early research into garlic's effect on lowering blood cholesterol, eight well-controlled trials have shown no improvement in people taking garlic for six months. More than two dozen studies examining garlic's effect on blood pressure also came up 'empty'.

It's a similar story for coenzyme Q10, a vitamin-like, fat-soluble substance. Trials examining its effects on heart failure patients have shown no benefits. Neither have trials looking at coenzyme Q10 for treatment of angina or hypertension.

Hawthorne root has been recommended for treatment of heart disease in many herbal medicine books. It has even been approved for heart failure patients in Germany and is marketed as a prescription drug there. But the clinical evidence for hawthorne root is less than astounding. In one look at eight studies with a total of some 600 patients, all of whom had congestive heart failure, the only plus to taking hawthorne root appeared to be an ability to exercise longer on a bicycle test and even that benefit has not been confirmed.

More important, hawthorne root and other complementary treatments have some potentially serious side effects. Hawthorne root can cause nausea, fatigue, sweating, palpitations and agitation. Coenzyme

Q10 can potentially interact with other drugs. Other substances that some people take to protect their hearts, such as the herb ginkgo biloba, can interfere with blood coagulation, which could be a very serious problem should you bleed as the result of an accident or have to undergo surgery, where bleeding is an expected part of the procedure.

Furthermore, while as many as 75 per cent of Americans take some kind of complementary or alternative substance, as few as 17 per cent tell their doctors about it. And that leaves doctors in the dark – and patients at risk for serious interactions between drugs that the doctors prescribe and over-the-counter herbs and other substances that the patients decide to take on their own.

If you want to try an over-the-counter preparation to help your heart, discuss it with your doctor, even if you think he or she will pooh-pooh your decision. What may seem like only trying to avoid a lecture about wasting your money could actually be a way of avoiding the use of your body as a site for a very dangerous science experiment.

of the stress hormone cortisol. It also lowers blood pressure. In a study at Johns Hopkins University in the US, a group of people who practised tai chi lowered their systolic pressure by an average of 7 points – just 1 point less than a separate group who engaged in low-impact aerobic dance. Now new research from some of our colleagues at Tufts, in conjunction with investigators at McGill University, has found that tai chi is associated with improved cardiovascular function in general. That's what they found when they conducted a review of nearly fifty studies on tai chi published over the last twenty years.

The relaxing moves, or poses, of tai chi, which have names like White Crane Spreads Its Wings and Step Up to Seven Stars, emphasize balance, breathing and body awareness. The aim is always on slow, deep breathing and focusing your energy.

Your local YWCA or health club probably offers a tai chi class. There are also good tai chi videos that you can practise with at home. (See the Resources section at the back of the book.) Keep in mind that tai chi can be posturally demanding. Thus, if you have balance problems, say, because of a medication you are taking, you should speak with your instructor before signing up so your programme can be modified accordingly.

Yoga

While the research regarding yoga's direct effects on heart health is scant, there are many reasons to believe that it has a beneficial effect. It is well accepted that in addition to improving physical fitness, yoga increases the mind's capacity for meditation. And since meditation relieves stress, which thereby helps the heart, it's fair to say that yoga is good for the heart.

Yoga often brings to mind people who contort themselves into pretzel-like poses while seeking spiritual enlightenment. Yet yoga is not just for the superflexible, double-jointed minority. Up to 10 million Americans currently engage in this ancient practice, which originated in India.

There are actually many types of yoga, but the kind most Americans think of is *hatha* yoga, which involves a variety of static postures, or *asanas.* Concentrated breathing exercises, or *pranayamas,* are involved, too.

Your local YWCA or health club is a good place to try on yoga for size by taking a class. Look for an instructor with several years' experience and make sure her or his style feels right to you. The governing body for yoga in the UK is the British Wheel of Yoga who have qualified teachers, see Resources.

Optimism

Optimism may not seem like something you can *do,* like yoga or tai chi. But it actually is possible to cultivate optimism, which can break the cycle of depression and thereby improve heart health. (Yes, optimistic people have less heart disease than pessimists.)

How? By disputing negative thoughts – literally. Let's say the pessimistic thought 'I'll never be able to lose weight' keeps running through your mind. Is that factually correct or just an over-reaction? Consider the evidence before you decide. Were there times in the past when you were able to reach a difficult goal? The answer is probably yes.

Also, instead of blaming yourself, as pessimistic thinkers tend to do, go over all the contributing factors to the situation and work through how they might be overcome. Is it really a matter of your not being able to stick with a plan, or is it that you actually stick very well to your plans but simply have many competing commitments right now and are having a hard time finding the emotional energy to fit in one more thing? Answering that question honestly will free you up to begin making some changes towards your goal rather than keep you stuck in the erroneous belief that you're simply not capable.

Pessimists can also brighten their outlook by writing things down. When you put your stress outside of yourself by keeping a journal, it's easier to look at your situation objectively and see where you're being held back rather than just assuming nothing will ever get better and the ball is out of your hands. It's not.

Social Outreach

Social isolation is one of the worst things for stress and depression. It gives negativity every opportunity to fester – and worm its way into your heart, both figuratively and literally. Indeed, research has shown that depressed people who live alone or have little contact with friends and relatives are at greater risk for death after a heart attack than depressed people who have a good social support network. Furthermore, people with only a small network of family and friends have a two- to threefold greater risk for developing heart disease over time than others.

If you have been socially isolated, the thought of 'getting out there' may seem overwhelming. One option is to find a walking partner. It fosters friendship without forcing it and you'll get some exercise, too!

We also suggest volunteer work. It builds a social component into your life without putting the emphasis on socializing per se. That, in turn, assuages anxiety about getting together with other people. Yet it will work to extend your social contacts, put you back 'in the loop' and bring your mind to a better place – particularly worthy benefits if you've recently been widowed or divorced and therefore might be at increased risk for social isolation because of depression, or perhaps because you're feeling like 'a fifth wheel' around other couples you've always socialized with.

Volunteering opportunities abound. You can work for a political or social cause, serve food in a soup kitchen, mentor young people and so on. You can also inquire at your local schools, hospital, community centre, library or place of worship to see if volunteers are needed.

Talk It Out

Perhaps the most important key for reducing the mental stress in your life in order to protect your heart is to bring it up with your doctor. The vast majority of stressed and depressed patients never get treatment because they never seek it. And doctors don't ask about it. In fact, if you wait for your doctor to ask whether something is bothering you, you may wait forever because most doctors are not trained to talk to patients about their feelings. Yet ironically, the medical community is better equipped than ever to treat depression, anxiety and hostility.

Indeed, in a small study published several years ago, heart patients on standard diet regimens who also sought and got emotional help – either in the form of group therapy, instruction in relaxation techniques or stress management training – showed greater reductions in psychological distress. They were also able to lower their blood pressure, heart rate and blood cholesterol.

Your doctor might refer you to a group therapist or psychologist for one-on-one sessions. A doctor can also discuss with you prescription drugs for depression or anxiety. Sometimes even just expressing to your doctor that you have undue stress or depression gets the healing process under way.

Speaking of Your Place of Worship . . .

For hundreds of years, Western medicine has treated the body and the soul separately. But the pendulum appears to be swinging back. More and more medical schools are now offering classes on spirituality and medicine. It's not surprising. In a study of patients who had undergone open-heart surgery, those who reported that they drew strength and comfort from religion appeared to have better outcomes after surgery than those who didn't.

The faithful seem to recover from depression more quickly, too. In a look at almost 100 people who became depressed after a hospital stay, researchers at Duke University, USA, found that those who scored high on a test of religious beliefs and experience bounced back faster than others. Other research suggests that religious people are less likely to become depressed in the first place.

Still more research has shown that people who attend services at least once a week – or frequently pray or study the Bible at least once a day – have slightly lower blood pressure than those who aren't as religiously active.

Faith appears to affect health on a number of fronts. One is so-called sin avoidance. Religious people often live relatively healthy lives – no smoking or excessive drinking, for instance. Organized religion also increases one's social circle, which buffers the harmful effects of isolation, stress, anxiety and depression. And prayer itself can be akin to meditation: the repetition in prayer, such as occurs with going through the Catholic rosary or *davening* (a swaying movement during certain prayers in some forms of Judaism), can be compared to repeating a mantra and the quiet, contemplative mood can be relaxing and profound.

Of course, you can't just march into a church, synagogue or mosque and expect your heart to get healthier. Faith is deeply held and commitment to one's faith has a lot to do with its benefits.

The good news: you don't have to be devout or spiritually inclined to reap many of the benefits. Through meditation, social outreach, volunteering and plain old good, clean living, you're taking advantage of all the secular advantages religion affords. That is, by availing yourself of the approaches in this chapter, as well as in the chapters on nutrition and exercise, you'll be treating your body like a temple – and giving your heart (and soul) the 'nourishment' it needs.

PART 3

Beyond
Lifestyle

CHAPTER 9

Sorting Through the Medication Options

◆

I was so disappointed that despite all my efforts to bring down my blood pressure through lifestyle – giving up alcohol, eating more than five fruits and vegetables a day, going easy on the salt, walking or running five miles three times a week and strength training twice a week – I still had to go on medication to get it into line. And then the dose had to be doubled because it started to creep up again. But when I told my doctor how bad I felt about it, he reminded me that other people in my family got high blood pressure in their thirties and forties, whereas I was able to hold it off until I was fifty. 'That's really great,' he said. 'Your preventative lifestyle kept it at bay for much longer.' He was right. That made me feel better about it.

— Anne

When it comes to taking a drug to control the course of a disease, many women fall into one of two camps. One camp holds the position that resorting to a drug means they've failed in their efforts to control the disease on their own; they resist taking the medicine because they feel it would mean they've failed at strong-arming the problem and may even resort to spending a lot of money on unproven over-the-counter preparations. The other camp's perspective is that the drug will 'take care of the problem'. As long as the pill is popped, they're all set and don't have to pay attention to anything else.

Neither one of those attitudes has any place in heart disease treatment. While lifestyle changes are the first line of defense for decreasing blood cholesterol and blood pressure to reduce the risk for heart attacks and strokes, in no way should you misconstrue a prescription for a drug as licence to abandon your efforts to eat a heart-healthy diet and get adequate exercise. Both the US National Institutes of Health and the American Heart Association are quite clear that the best outcomes happen to those people who continue to protect their hearts through lifestyle changes as they follow through with a prescription. Reverting to a poor diet and a sedentary way of living – and letting your weight creep up – not only reduces the benefit, it can work against you by making it harder for the drug to do its job. Indeed, we have heard anecdotally that some people have been known to eat their way around a drug, making it difficult to control their blood cholesterol levels even though the drugs to keep down cholesterol are so powerful.

As for those who feel that resorting to a drug means that they couldn't 'cut it' and are officially sick, nothing could be further from the truth. Taking the right medication means you're taking advantage of the best twenty-first-century medicine has to offer to allow you to lead a full, productive life for a longer period of time and, indeed, to *save* your life. Consider that since the 1987 introduction of statin drugs, potent agents that lower blood cholesterol, people are living who absolutely would be dead otherwise. According to a large analysis, statins reduce heart disease risk by up to 60 per cent and stroke risk by up to 17 per cent.

And drugs to improve people's heart disease profile are getting better all the time. The pharmacologic gamut for heart-saving medications, in fact, is something of a moving target, with recommended drugs – and their dosages – changing as researchers continue to learn how to keep the cardiovascular system protected. For that reason, the list of drugs that follows should be thought of as a general guide (and by no means a complete one) to the current drug arsenal. Your doctor may very well tell you to take something not mentioned here, or she or he may adjust your dosage depending on such factors as what other drugs you are taking. It's okay to ask your doctor to explain her or his decision if it conflicts with what you read here or elsewhere, but in the end follow your doctor's directions. Your doctor has all the particulars on you and your body, which allows for the best tailoring of drugs and drug prescriptions.

DRUGS THAT LOWER LDL-CHOLESTEROL

Medications for lowering cholesterol have undergone an amazing metamorphosis over the last twenty years and even the last ten. To say that the arsenal of cholesterol lowerers today wasn't available when your mother was your age is a vast understatement. Sometimes two drugs with different modes of action are prescribed simultaneously for maximum effect.

Statins

With statins having changed the face of heart disease treatment and heart disease being the biggest killer of American women as well as men, it should come as no surprise that statins are now the largest selling class of prescription medications in the United States, ahead of antidepressants, anti-heartburn agents, even pills for high blood pressure.

There are six statin drugs altogether, with more on the way. Here are their names:

- lovastatin (Mevacor)
- simastatin (Zocor)
- fluvastatin (Lescol)
- atorvastatin (Lipitor)
- pravastatin (Lipostat)
- rosuvastatin (Crestor)

MODE OF ACTION: All statins work in a similar way. They inhibit cells in the liver and elsewhere from making cholesterol. That forces these cells to pull cholesterol out of the bloodstream, reducing circulating levels.

EFFICACY: People who take statins typically undergo a 20 to 60 per cent reduction in LDL-cholesterol. Statins also (modestly) reduce elevated triglycerides and (modestly) increase HDL-cholesterol.

PRESCRIPTION DIRECTIONS: Some people are told to take statins with the evening meal or at bedtime. The body tends to produce more cholesterol at night than during the day. After four to eight weeks, blood cholesterol is re-evaluated and the prescription adjusted, if necessary.

SIDE EFFECTS: In general, statins are very well tolerated, with a low rate of side effects. Occasionally reported are stomach upset, gas, constipation and abdominal cramps. Fortunately, these gastrointestinal symptoms often abate with time.

More rare side effects include abnormal elevations in blood liver enzymes and muscle aches and pains. Most of the time, the rise in blood liver enzymes doesn't have any practical significance. It's reversible; the enzyme levels drop either with a lower dose or by switching to another statin.

The muscle aches and pains occur in 4 to 5 per cent of people who go on statins. Sometimes they get better on their own, but they can also get worse. The effects on muscle are particularly an issue for older women.

Your doctor can sometimes correct a side-effect problem by lowering the dose or switching you to another statin. In extremely rare cases, a different class of cholesterol-lowering drug may be called for.

Resins, Also Known as Bile Acid Sequestrants

Resins were developed long before statins became available and are sometimes added to the treatment regimen if statins alone aren't doing the trick. But they don't tend to be used much anymore. They can be poorly tolerated – they have an unpleasant mouth feel and may cause constipation and bloating. For these reasons, compliance is low. There are three resin drugs:

- cholestyramine (Questran)
- colestipol (Colestid)
- colesevelam (Cholestagel)

MODE OF ACTION: Resins do their work in the lower part of the intestine. Specifically, they bind bile acids to them, forcing them to be excreted in the stools. Why is that important? Bile acids (which are essential for dietary fat diges-

The Cause of High Cholesterol Isn't Always What You Think It Is

High cholesterol doesn't always stem from the usual culprits. In some heart disease clinics, about 5 to 10 per cent of patients who have been referred by their general practictioners actually have an underactive thyroid, which is not an uncommon cause of high cholesterol in itself. Usually, they're elderly and often, they're women.

To lower their cholesterol, their general practitioner has prescribed a statin (after suggesting changes in diet and physical activity), but it doesn't work (and may also cause statins' telltale side effects) because the problem has an unrelated cause. So the doctor sends these patients to a heart specialist to get to the bottom of what seems like an intractable problem.

A savvy doctor, however, will check a woman's thyroid before referring her to a cardiologist – particularly if she brings up that she has been feeling fatigued lately, cannot tolerate cold as well as usual and perhaps has been constipated. These are all possible signs of a thyroid problem. If an underactive thyroid is indeed diagnosed (which is often the case), the patient is given thyroid hormone and *voilà*, blood cholesterol drops into the healthy range. The woman also feels a lot better all of a sudden – less fatigued, less cold and less constipated.

tion and absorption) are made from cholesterol in the liver. Excrete them and you force your liver to take up more cholesterol from the bloodstream in order to replace the bile acids that have been lost.

EFFICACY: Resins tend to lower LDL-cholesterol by 10 to 20 per cent.

PRESCRIPTION DIRECTIONS: Resins come in powder or tablet form. They must be mixed with water or fruit juice and taken once or twice a day, with meals. Taking them with adequate fluids is important to avoid constipation, as is taking them with food to minimize side effects.

SIDE EFFECTS: Primarily gastrointestinal in nature, side effects include constipation, bloating, nausea, gas and worsening of haemorrhoids.

Nicotinic Acid or Niacin (Niacor)

Nicotinic acid, or niacin, is actually one of the B vitamins. But whereas the amount for general dietary adequacy for women is 14 milligrams per day, it takes thousands of milligrams (2 to 3 grams) for niacin to lower cholesterol.

Because nicotinic acid is a nutrient, it's available over the counter as a dietary supplement. However, for the purpose of reducing elevated cholesterol, it should be taken *only* under the direction of a doctor. We cannot stress this enough. Side effects can be significant and must be carefully monitored by a doctor.

There are two types of nicotinic acid (not to be confused with nicotinamide, which is also a form of niacin but cannot lower blood cholesterol):

- immediate release
- timed/extended release

MODE OF ACTION: Nicotinic acid decreases production of particles in the liver that are necessary for carrying cholesterol and fat in the bloodstream.

EFFICACY: This drug lowers LDL-cholesterol by 10 to 20 per cent. It also lowers triglycerides – by 20 to 50 per cent. And it raises the HDL-cholesterol concentration by 15 to 35 per cent.

PRESCRIPTION DIRECTIONS: People are usually started on the immediate-release form. To minimize side effects, doses often begin on the relatively low side and are gradually increased to anywhere from 1.5 to 3 grams a day. If timed- or extended-release forms are used, the dose usually tops out at 1.5 to 2.0 grams daily.

SIDE EFFECTS: There are several potential side effects. One is flushing or hot flushes – a result of blood vessels suddenly opening up. Some patients develop a tolerance for the hot flushes. Others can minimize the flushing by taking the drug with meals or aspirin (under the guidance of a doctor). Timed/extended-release forms result in less flushing in some but not all people.

There can also be an increased effect of certain blood pressure medications. In some cases, nicotinic acid and blood pressure medication taken together can make blood pressure fall too low. The use of such medications must be coordinated by your doctor.

Other possibilities include GI upset and an increase in liver enzymes that could signify liver dysfunction, high blood sugar (which is why it's not generally recommended for people with diabetes) and gout, which is a form of arthritis.

Ezetimibe (Ezetrol)

Ezetimibe, a relatively new drug, is most commonly used as an adjunct to statins when statin treatment alone is not enough to bring cholesterol levels into the desired range.

MODE OF ACTION: Whereas statins inhibit cholesterol production, ezetimibe decreases cholesterol *absorption* from the small intestine.

EFFICACY: This drug decreases LDL-cholesterol an average of 12 per cent over and above what statins alone will do.

PRESCRIPTION DIRECTIONS: Ezetimibe comes in tablet form and should be taken once a day with meals or at the same time you take a statin.

SIDE EFFECTS: Adverse effects are primarily gastrointestinal and include constipation, bloating, nausea and gas.

Plant Sterols

Naturally occurring compounds isolated from tree bark, soya beans or other sources, plant sterols are added to certain foods – some margarine and yogurts, for example. They also come in softgel capsules. They are used to lower cholesterol to some degree in Finland but haven't really caught on in other countries. In this country, some people seem to be hesitant about consuming foods manufactured with the express purpose of having a pharmacological effect.

MODE OF ACTION: Plant sterols are thought to inhibit cholesterol absorption.

EFFICACY: They lower LDL-cholesterol by 10 to15 per cent.

PRESCRIPTION DIRECTIONS: The average amount recommended is 1.6 to 2.0 grams a day. Levels vary among products – you may need four servings of margarine, for instance – so if you and your doctor decide you should go the plant sterol route, you'll need to follow the directions on the label of the food(s) you're going to use.

Note: We are not particularly enamoured of the idea of putting drugs into foods, if for no other reason than once you add a food to the diet to lower cholesterol, you have to subtract calories somewhere else, so it is somewhat complicated. Also, because different foods contain different amounts of plant sterols, standardized dosing becomes difficult, if not impossible. That said, plant sterols are certainly a legitimate way to go; the US National Heart, Lung and Blood Institute has endorsed their use. If you're going to try them, we suggest you discuss with your doctor the advisability of using the softgel capsules.

SIDE EFFECTS: Generally well tolerated, plant sterols have been reported in rare cases to cause mild indigestion.

DRUGS THAT AFFECT OTHER LIPIDS

LDL-cholesterol is not the only blood lipid treated with drugs. There are also medications to raise HDL-cholesterol as well as lower triglycerides.

Fibrates

Fibrates lower elevated triglycerides. They may also raise HDL-cholesterol. (The two tend to go hand in hand.) The fibrates available are:

- gemfibrozil (Lopid)
- clofibrate (Atromid-S)
- fenofibrate (Lipantil, Tricor)

MODE OF ACTION: Fibrates operate by increasing the rate at which triglycerides are removed from VLDL, which stands for very low-density lipoprotein.

EFFICACY: The reduction in triglyceride levels ranges from 20 to 50 per cent. Elevations in HDL-cholesterol range from 10 to 15 per cent.

PRESCRIPTION DIRECTIONS: Fibrates are usually given in two daily doses, thirty minutes before the morning and evening meals.

SIDE EFFECTS: These drugs are well tolerated by most patients. The most common side effect, as with many of the others, is gastrointestinal discomfort. But fibrates can also elevate the risk of developing gallstones. And they may increase the potency of anticoagulants, sometimes referred to as blood thinners, making monitoring by a doctor essential.

Fish Oil Capsules

As we discussed in chapter 4, fish oil contains EPA and DHA, omega-3 fatty acids that help lower high triglycerides, make blood less 'sticky' by decreasing platelet aggregation and most important, decrease the risk of sudden cardiac death. For these reasons, as we discussed in chapter 5, everyone should be aiming for at least two fish meals a week. But some doctors advise people who have had a heart attack to take fish oil *capsules,* which have higher doses of fish oil than fish itself. Milk containing omega-3 fatty acids is also available now in supermarkets, produced by cows which are given a special fish oil blend in their feed. It tastes the same as ordinary milk but provides 10 times more of the acids DHA and EPA than regular milk.

MODE OF ACTION: All the various ways in which fish oil decreases heart disease risk are not known, but researchers are aware that fish oil capsules decrease the incidence of arrhythmias and blood clotting.

EFFICACY: Three to four grams or so of fish oil a day (more than you could get in four or five fish meals) decrease triglycerides 25 to 30 per cent. About

1 gram a day has been shown to decrease future heart attack risk in people who have already had a heart attack. Doctors decide how much to prescribe based on a patient's individual history.

PRESCRIPTION DIRECTIONS: While fish oil capsules are available over the counter, they should be taken only under a doctor's supervision. One reason is that while they lower triglycerides, they can also *increase* LDL-cholesterol up to 10 per cent, so anyone who takes them has to be monitored.

SIDE EFFECTS: Adverse effects, which occur at levels greater than 1 gram a day, are primarily gastrointestinal in nature and include constipation, bloating, nausea, fishy belches and gas. Excess amounts can make you prone to bleeding in the case of an accident or emergency surgery.

Does a Baby Aspirin a Day Keep the Doctor Away?

A lot of men are told by their doctors to take baby, or low-dose, aspirin regularly in order to prevent heart disease. Should women? It depends on your heart disease risk, says the American Heart Association. Given the lack of definitive evidence in women, it also depends on your doctor's assessment of your particular situation. You should not buy it over the counter without her or his recommendation. Aspirin can cause gastrointestinal bleeding and the risk of that has to be weighed against the benefit to your heart.

ASPIRIN THERAPY FOR WOMEN

at high risk:	75–162 milligrams a day* (1 to 2 baby aspirin)
at intermediate risk:	75–162 milligrams a day*
at low risk:	not recommended

While the dose is the same for high and intermediate risk, a doctor's decision to prescribe aspirin will depend on a woman's individual risk for side effects.

DRUGS THAT LOWER BLOOD PRESSURE

In more than two out of three people with hypertension, the condition cannot be controlled with one drug alone. Note that there are far more antihypertensive medications than drugs for cholesterol. In addition, they are frequently prescribed and sold in combination. We provide here information on general classes.

Diuretics

Diuretics, referred to by some people as 'water pills', are usually the first drug of choice for people who cannot control their blood pressure through diet and exercise alone. The three major types of diuretics are thiazides, loop diuretics and potassium-sparing diuretics.

1. Thiazides (also known as potassium-depleting diuretics)

Examples:

- chlorothiazide (Diuril and others)
- hydrochlorothiazide (Esidrix, Hydrodiuril)
- polythiazide (Nephril)
- indapamide (Natrilix)
- metolazone (Mykrox, Zaroxolyn, Metenix)

2. Loop diuretics (also known as potassium-depleting diuretics). These are more potent than thiazide diuretics. In addition to lowering blood pressure, they are the most effective in reducing the amount of fluid volume in the body, which is good for people with congestive heart failure.

Examples:

- bumetanide (Burinex)
- furosemide (Lasix and others)
- torsemide (Torem)

3. Potassium-sparing diuretics

Examples:

- amiloride (Amil-Co)
- triamterene (Dytac)

MODE OF ACTION: Diuretics cause the body to rid itself of excess fluids (and sodium) through urination. When there is less fluid volume in the vascular system, there is less pressure on artery walls as blood is pumped through all the blood vessels. That is, the pressure of blood in the arteries is reduced.

EFFICACY: Varies from drug to drug and patient to patient.

PRESCRIPTION DIRECTIONS: Sometimes, the recommendation for those taking potassium-depleting diuretics is to eat potassium-rich foods (see page 67 for examples). In other instances the doctor may prescribe supplemental potassium. If you miss a dose of a diuretic, wait until the next time. Do not take the dose late or double up. Diuretics should be stored at room temperature, away from moisture, light and excess heat.

SIDE EFFECTS: Potassium-sparing diuretics can cause weakness, leg cramps or fatigue if body potassium runs too low. But generally diuretics tend to be well tolerated (although there have been some reports of sexual dysfunction and urinary incontinence).

Angiotensin-Converting Enzyme (ACE Inhibitors)

ACE inhibitors not only can lower blood pressure but also are used to treat heart failure. Some common ACE inhibitors include:

- benazepril (Lotrel)
- captopril (Capoten, Acepril)
- enalapril (Innovace)
- fosinopril (Staril)
- lisinopril (Carace, Zestril)
- moexipril (Perdix)

- perindopril (Coversyl)
- quinapril (Accupro)
- ramipril (Tritace)
- trandolapril (Gopten, Odrik)

MODE OF ACTION: ACE inhibitors prevent the formation of a hormone called *angiotensin II,* which causes blood vessels to narrow. By 'relaxing' the blood vessels, it actually allows them to expand as blood is forced out of the heart, thereby decreasing resistance to blood flowing through them. That, in turn, lowers the pressure of the blood on the artery walls. Of course, that also makes the heart's pumping work easier and more efficient. It doesn't have to pump as hard to push blood through all the arteries.

EFFICACY: Varies from drug to drug and patient to patient.

PRESCRIPTION DIRECTIONS: If you miss a dose, wait until the next time. Do not take the dose late or double up. Store at room temperature, away from moisture, light and excess heat.

SIDE EFFECTS: Potential adverse effects, which are rare, include cough, skin rash, loss of taste and compromised renal function. ACE inhibitors should be avoided by pregnant women.

Angiotensin II Receptor Antagonists

Angiotensin II receptor antagonists have been shown to produce blood pressure lowering effects similar to those produced by ACE inhibitors. Current angiotensin II receptor antagonists include:

- candesartan (Amias)
- eprosartan (Teveten)
- irbesartan (Aprovel)
- losartan (Cozaar)
- olmesartan (Olmetec)
- telmisartan (Micardis)
- valsartan (Diovan)

MODE OF ACTION: Whereas ACE inhibitors lower levels of angiotensin II, angiotensin II receptor antagonists prevent the blood vessel constricting hormone from acting on cells that line the surface of blood vessels. They can be thought to 'shield' blood vessels from angiotensin II.

EFFICACY: Varies from drug to drug and patient to patient.

PRESCRIPTION DIRECTIONS: If you miss a dose, wait until next time. Do not take the dose late or double up. Store at room temperature, away from moisture, light and excess heat.

SIDE EFFECTS: Some people occasionally experience dizziness. Angiotensin II receptor antagonists should be avoided by pregnant women.

Beta-Blockers

In addition to being used to lower blood pressure, beta-blockers are sometimes prescribed to treat cardiac arrhythmias and angina and can also be useful for patients with congestive heart failure. Current beta-blockers include:

- acebutolol (Sectral)
- atenolol (Tenormin)
- betaxolol (Betoptic)
- bisoprolol (Cardicor, Emcor, Monocor)
- metoprolol (Lopresor, Betaloc)
- nadolol (Corgard)
- propranolol (Inderal)
- propranolol long-acting (Beta-prograne)
- timolol (Nyogel, Timoptol)

MODE OF ACTION: Beta-blockers decrease heart rate. That means that both the intervals between each pump of blood last a little longer and the heart pumps a little less intensely, cutting down on how often – and how much – pressure is exerted on the arteries as blood rushes through them.

EFFICACY: Varies from drug to drug and patient to patient.

PRESCRIPTION DIRECTIONS: If you miss a dose, wait until next time. Do not take two doses close together or double up. Store at room temperature, away from moisture, light and excess heat.

SIDE EFFECTS: Dizziness, fatigue, insomnia, cold hands and feet and depression have been reported, but these medications are usually well tolerated.

Calcium Channel Blockers

In addition to controlling high blood pressure, calcium channel blockers are used to treat angina and some arrhythmias. Current channel blockers on the market include:

- amlodipine (Istin)
- diltiazem extended release (Adizem, Angitil SR, Dilzem and others)
- felodipine (Plendil)
- isradipine (Prescal)
- nicardipine sustained release (Cardene SR)
- nifedipine long acting (Fortipine LA)
- nisoldipine (Syscor MR)
- verapamil long acting (Vertab SR)
- verapamil (Cordilox, Securon, Univer, Zolvera)

MODE OF ACTION: Also known as calcium antagonists, calcium channel blockers interrupt the movement of the mineral calcium into cardiovascular cells. That causes the blood vessels to relax, which makes for less resistance; hence, there is less pressure on the artery walls as blood rushes through.

EFFICACY: Varies from drug to drug and patient to patient.

PRESCRIPTION DIRECTIONS: Take as directed. If you skip a dose, wait until next time. Do not take two doses close together or double up. Store at room temperature, away from moisture, light and excess heat.

SIDE EFFECTS: They differ widely among drugs. Constipation, swollen ankles, headache and dizziness are some of the more common ones.

BE SMART: LISTEN TO YOUR DOCTOR

As you can see, the arsenal of drugs available to treat cholesterol levels, other lipids and blood pressure is enormous – and keeps getting bigger and more effective all the time. Every year, new medications reach the market.

The unfortunate truth is that not enough women are *taking* them. For example, three out of four women with high blood pressure are aware of it, but fewer than one in three are taking the necessary steps to control it. If your doctor determines that a prescription is necessary, take the drug faithfully to live as long and as healthily as possible. Comments Anne, who got her high blood pressure under control with medication, 'I have a twenty-one-year-old, a seventeen-year-old and an eleven-year-old. I fully intend to be in their lives for quite a while.'

CHAPTER 10

Angioplasty, Bypass, Cardiac Catheterization: The ABCs of Medical Procedures

◆

I woke up in the middle of the night, sweating. I couldn't breathe. I called 999. When I got to the hospital, the doctor said I had had a heart attack. They did an angioplasty right then and there and put three stents in three different places to open my arteries. I had heard the term 'angioplasty', but I never knew what it was. I was awake during the procedure – and scared. If I had known before about all of this, I would have had less anxiety.

— PEARL

There are times when, no matter what you do for your heart lifestyle-wise, you end up having to go through a heart-related procedure. Sometimes it's surgery; more often, it's simply a diagnostic test. Either way, it can be very scary. Tubes, anaesthesia, complicated machinery and other unfamiliar medical devices and, today, staff that may not have enough time to really explain what is happening and answer all your questions – all of that can produce a lot of anxiety on top of the anxiety a woman is already feeling if a doctor says she needs some kind of invasive test or operation.

But just knowing what it is you're being put through, for exactly what heart-saving reason, can greatly decrease the fear and anxiety about undergoing a new procedure.

What follows are some of the most common procedures – both diagnostic procedures and treatment procedures – related to the heart, including what they entail and how they help. (Similar procedures are used to predict stroke risk.) Should you end up needing one of them, you can consult this book ahead of time. Knowledge isn't just power. It's also reassurance.

Please note that procedures differ to some degree from hospital to hospital and also are being updated all the time, so the way things go may not always be exactly the way they are described here. But the explanations will serve as a reasonable resource; you will not feel in the dark should one of these tests or operations be recommended.

DIAGNOSTIC PROCEDURES FOR CORONARY ARTERY DISEASE

Many of the diagnostic procedures listed below allow a doctor to 'see' the heart or arteries – or the blood flowing through them – without actually opening you up. That is, what previously would have needed to be done with an operation can now be done with less invasive approaches.

Prior to the start of many of these procedures, risks for complications (which are very rare) will be explained. (Some people have reactions to the dyes used to see an artery during an imaging technique, for instance.) You may also be asked to sign a witnessed consent form.

Cardiac Catheterization/Coronary Angiography

If you're feeling chest pain upon even light exertion such as walking up the stairs, your doctor may send you for this procedure. It provides information on blood pressure within the heart; how much oxygen is in the blood flowing through the heart and coronary arteries; and the heart's pumping ability. Cardiac catheterization is often performed in tandem with coronary angioplasty (see page 195).

HOW IT WORKS: First, an intravenous line is inserted into a blood vessel through either the groin or an arm. Then, under the guidance of X-rays, a catheter, or thin tube, is inserted right through the intravenous line to the location in the heart or blood vessel that's of interest (that's the catheterization part). Next, a dye is inserted into the catheter (the angiography part). Because it's of a colour-contrast material, the dye is visible with X-rays and thereby gives an indication of whether, or to what degree, your blood is flowing, or more important, *where* blood flow is impeded or partially blocked. For instance, it can show how much of an artery's diameter is closed off due to plaque or other blockages.

BEFORE THE PROCEDURE: Usually, you will be told to restrict food and fluid for a period of time before the test.

About thirty minutes prior to the catheterization, you may be given a mild sedative. You'll also be told to lie flat on your back and the area where the catheter will be inserted will be cleansed. A local anaesthetic will be used to numb the site where the IV will be inserted.

DURING THE PROCEDURE: You will be awake throughout the procedure. Because blood vessels do not have nerve endings, it is unlikely that you will feel the catheter while the angiography is being performed. You may simply feel some pressure at the site where the catheter is inserted and, since the procedure can last from one to several hours, you may feel some discomfort from having to remain in one position for that length of time.

AFTER THE PROCEDURE: When the catheter is removed, firm pressure will be applied at the site of insertion to prevent bleeding. If the catheter was inserted in the groin, you will likely be asked to remain lying on your back for a few hours after the procedure to avoid bleeding.

Electrocardiogram (ECG, EKG)

An electrocardiogram measures the electrical activity of the heart, which allows for an assessment of the heart rate and the regularity of heartbeats. It can also assess the size of the heart chambers, the presence of any damage to the heart muscle and the effects of drugs or devices used to regulate the heart.

HOW IT WORKS The doctor or doctor's assistant will affix electrodes – little disks – to your arms, legs and chest while you are in the reclining position. The number of electrodes varies, ranging from as few as three to five to as many as twelve to fifteen. The electrodes measure the heart's electrical activity, which allows for an assessment of electric pulsations associated with the heart's squeezing, or pumping, function. The measurements are indicated with a series of blips on a long line inked onto a piece of paper or imaged on a computer screen. Different patterns or intervals in those blips indicate how long electrical waves take to pass from one part of the heart to the other. Read by trained personnel, the patterns provide information on how your heart is functioning.

BEFORE THE PROCEDURE: There are no restrictions on consumption of food or medications prior to this procedure. Simply, the areas where the electrodes will be placed will be cleansed.

DURING THE PROCEDURE: You may feel a little cold at the sites where the disks are attached. You will not feel anything else since the ECG machine to which the electrodes are attached is only measuring electrical impulses normally going through your heart. The whole procedure takes about five minutes.

AFTER THE PROCEDURE: In rare circumstances, a rash or irritation may develop at the sites where the disks were attached.

Echocardiogram (Transthoracic Echocardiogram; Doppler Ultrasound of the Heart)

An echocardiogram is an ultrasound of the heart, meaning that sound waves are used to create a two-dimensional picture of the heart muscle as it pumps and squeezes. (Think of how an ultrasound allows a developing foetus to be seen as it moves about in the uterus.) The picture, which is much more detailed than what an X-ray could provide, allows a doctor (usually a cardiologist) to view the valves, walls and chambers of the heart in a non-invasive manner. It also allows assessment of movement to evaluate pumping capacity or flow characteristics. Specifically, echocardiograms allow doctors to assess heart murmurs, check the pumping strength and efficiency of the heart and check up on patients who have had a heart attack.

HOW IT WORKS: An instrument called a transducer is placed on various spots on the chest and directed towards the heart. The transducer sends out high-frequency sound waves and then picks up their echoes, which will change based on the heart's structure and function. It then transmits the echoes as electrical impulses to a computerized echocardiography machine that converts them into actual pictures of the heart.

BEFORE THE PROCEDURE: No special preparation is required.

DURING THE PROCEDURE: No dyes or X-rays are involved. A gel will be spread on your chest and the transducer will then be applied. You will feel a slight pressure from the transducer but nothing else. You may be asked to breathe in a certain way or to roll over onto your left side.

AFTER THE PROCEDURE: You should feel no different from before the procedure.

Exercise Stress Test

An exercise stress test assesses the effect of exercise on your heart. In some cases, it may be ordered by your doctor when you talk to her or him about starting an exercise programme. More often, it is performed to determine whether you have blockages in the arteries supplying your heart, to determine your exercise capacity or to identify heart rate rhythm disturbances during exercise.

Often, the heart is imaged both just before and during or immediately after a stress test, which strengthens diagnostic accuracy. This is particularly important for women, who tend to have higher episodes of false positives on standard stress tests than men. Imaging is generally done with either echocardiography or what is known as nuclear scanning. Sometimes with echocardiography but always with nuclear scanning, an IV is inserted in the arm before exercise begins and special substances infused that facilitate imaging of the blood supplying the heart as well as the heart's pumping action.

HOW IT WORKS: Essentially, an electrocardiogram is performed while you walk (or run) on a treadmill or pedal on a stationary bicycle. These conditions are intended to simulate a situation in which your heart needs to respond to the demand for extra oxygen.

BEFORE THE PROCEDURE: Your doctor or hospital will give you instructions, which frequently involve not eating or drinking for about three hours before the test. Wear comfortable, loose-fitting clothing and appropriate shoes. Electrodes will be attached to your chest, arms and legs. A blood pressure cuff will be placed around one arm.

DURING THE PROCEDURE: You will be asked to walk, run or pedal, usually until you reach a target heart rate or you can't continue because you are too tired. Your heart rate and blood pressure will be monitored throughout the procedure. Sometimes, if you experience chest pain or your blood pressure increases precipitously during the test, you will be told to stop.

AFTER THE PROCEDURE: Heart rate and blood pressure are usually monitored for ten to fifteen minutes after you complete the exercise. You will likely feel the blood pressure cuff inflate and deflate at regular intervals.

Besides possibly feeling a little tired, you should not feel any different after you complete a stress test. In rare circumstances, a rash or irritation may develop at the sites where the disks were attached.

Myocardial Biopsy

A myocardial biopsy is often performed if cardiomyopathy (inflammation of the heart muscle) or cardiac amyloidosis (deposition of abnormal proteins in the heart muscle) is suspected. It's also conducted after a heart transplant to detect potential rejection of the new heart tissue.

HOW IT WORKS: Small pieces of heart muscle (usually three to five) are removed for examination.

BEFORE THE PROCEDURE: Several days before the test, you will likely be told to stop taking aspirin or other medications that affect bleeding time. You will be asked to restrict food and fluid intake for six to eight hours before the procedure. A mild sedative will be given to you about thirty minutes before the biopsy takes place. You will be asked to lie flat on your back. Local anaesthesia will be applied at the spot where a catheter will be inserted.

DURING THE PROCEDURE: As with a cardiac catheterization, you will be awake throughout. If cardiac tissue is needed from the right ventricle, a catheter is inserted through a vein (usually the jugular vein in the neck, sometimes with X-rays to guide the catheter). If it's needed from the left ventricle, it's inserted through an artery. Either way, a jaw-like apparatus on the tip of the catheter is used to snip off small pieces of heart muscle tissue.

AFTER THE PROCEDURE: You will have some pressure applied to the site where the catheter was inserted in order to prevent bleeding.

TREATMENT PROCEDURES

All of these procedures require admittance to the hospital, either as a day-patient or as an in-patient. Leave all your jewellery (including rings, if possible) and other valuables at home. You will be asked to sign a witnessed consent form to acknowledge your understanding that there are rare cases of complications.

Angioplasty (Balloon Angioplasty)

Angioplasty is performed to widen a blood vessel that has been narrowed, or blocked, by atherosclerotic plaque. The blockage is often discovered during a coronary angiography and the angioplasty (often in tandem with a cardiac catheterization) is performed right then, with the aim of increasing blood flow to the compromised area. The end result is relief from chest pain and improved exercise capacity.

HOW IT WORKS: A catheter with an inflatable balloon at the tip is inserted into the narrowed artery. It is then positioned right in or near the atherosclerotic blockage and inflated, which widens the blood vessel and restores adequate blood flow.

BEFORE THE PROCEDURE: Usually, you will be told to restrict food and fluid for a period of time before the test. About thirty minutes prior to the catheterization, you may be given a mild sedative. You'll also be told to lie flat on your back and the area where the catheter will be inserted will be cleansed. A local anaesthetic will be given to numb the site and the catheter will then be inserted (usually near the groin but sometimes in the arm or even the neck).

DURING THE PROCEDURE: An antiplatelet drug will be administered to minimize the risk of forming a blood clot. As the blocked blood vessel is opened and blood starts flowing smoothly once again, a *stent*, which is nothing more than a wire-mesh tube, is sometimes placed at the site as a kind of scaffolding to ensure that the area remains open. It remains in place permanently.

AFTER THE PROCEDURE: Pressure will be applied to the site where the catheter was inserted to avoid bleeding. You will have to lie still for several hours to allow the blood vessels at the point of entry to seal completely. The area may remain sore for up to one week, although you will usually leave the hospital the next day or the day after. When you are discharged, you will be given guidelines on what you may and may not do once you return home.

Angioplasty Variations

Percutaneous Transmyocardial Coronary Angioplasty (Transmyocardial Revascularization)

This procedure is usually performed to relieve severe angina or chest pain in very ill patients who aren't candidates for bypass surgery or traditional angioplasty. A surgeon makes an incision in the breast, exposing the heart. With a laser, she or he then drills several small holes into the heart's pumping chamber. How this procedure helps is unclear. It may be that the laser stimulates the growth of new blood vessels by causing bleeding. Another theory is that the laser destroys nerve fibres to the heart, which could reduce pain.

Laser Angioplasty

This treatment is not widely available in the UK, but depending on where you live and where your doctor is prepared to refer you, can can get it on the NHS; other techniques are seen as more effective. Once in place at or near the blockage, the laser emits pulsating beams of light that vaporize the plaque.

Bypass Surgery

If a blockage in an artery is severe or if blockages are too widespread for angioplasty and stenting, coronary artery bypass surgery will likely be necessary. Women who undergo bypass surgery sometimes have angina prior to the operation; that is what brings them in to see their doctor. They may have a feeling of heaviness, tightness, pain, pressure, squeezing or any of the most general symptoms of a heart attack. However, symptoms in women are often subtle and only diagnostic testing leads to the discovery of disease advanced enough to require the surgery.

BLOCKED ARTERY

BYPASS

Bypass surgery: A vein from a breast or leg is grafted onto a coronary artery above and below the blockage.

HOW IT WORKS: Also known as a coronary artery bypass graft, or CABG, by-pass surgery is just that. It uses a blood vessel from the leg or chest to by-pass (go around) a coronary artery that is blocked by atherosclerotic plaque. That allows the heart muscle to be nourished with blood it was otherwise deprived of.

BEFORE THE PROCEDURE: Because you will be under general anaesthesia, you will be instructed not to eat or drink for eight to twelve hours before the surgery.

DURING THE PROCEDURE: The traditional approach during bypass has been for the patient to be connected to a heart-lung machine that does the work of those two organs for the duration of the operation; the heart's beating is temporarily stopped while blood flows through the machine instead. But that creates potential complications in the way of declines in memory and mental clarity, lung and kidney complications and an increased risk for stroke. A newer approach, called *off-pump coronary artery bypass* or simply *minimally invasive heart surgery* (see below), allows the heart to keep pumping during the surgery and also avoids opening the chest.

AFTER THE PROCEDURE: Heart rate and blood pressure will be monitored con-tinuously for twelve to twenty-four hours. A urinary catheter and IV will remain in place until you're stable. An endotracheal tube will also stay in place until you are awake and can breathe comfortably on your own.

The incision in the chest and graft sites will be uncomfortable for forty-eight to seventy-two hours. You will be provided painkillers as needed.

You may spend three to five days in the hospital, with the first couple of hours in intensive care. You may have some 'fuzzy thinking' during that time.

A cardiac rehabilitation programme should begin when your doctor, in consultation with you, feels it's appropriate – sometimes while you're in the hospital but often after you return home.

When you do get back home, you may have loss of appetite, constipation, swelling at areas of incision, fatigue, mood swings and difficulty sleeping. These side effects, which don't affect everybody, can last four to six weeks. Usually, you can resume sexual activity four weeks after the surgery and return to work in four to six weeks. The full benefits of the operation can take as long as three to six months to be realized, although sometimes sooner. Many people report feeling much better than they have in years.

Bypass Variation: Minimally Invasive Heart Surgery

With this type of bypass, the heart continues beating during the operation. This allows the procedure to be performed without a heart-lung machine, making the operation safer than traditional bypass surgery. The patient tends to require fewer blood transfusions, has a decreased risk of stroke, a shorter postoperative hospital stay and a shorter recovery period. There are two main types:

Minimally Invasive Direct Coronary Bypass

This is for blockages in a coronary artery located in the front of the heart. A small incision (2 to 4 inches) is made in the left chest before the procedure is performed.

Off-Pump Coronary Artery Bypass

A vertical incision the size of the incision for traditional bypass surgery is made in the chest and the breastbone is split to allow access to the entire heart. A stabilizing device is put over the section of the beating heart to restrict movement where the blockage will be bypassed.

Heart Valve Surgery

As you'll recall from chapter 2, heart valves keep blood flowing in the right direction through the heart's chambers. But they need to be repaired or replaced if they leak blood backward (*regurgitation*) or become too narrow to let sufficient blood pass (*stenosis*). Defective valves that are not dealt with may cause congestive heart failure. Heart valve problems can originate in a number of ways: via infections, such as rheumatic fever; birth defects; calcification (hardening of the actual valve); or from certain medications (the weight-loss drug combination Fen-Phen, for example).

Save Someone *Else's* Life

Nearly everyone is familiar with the crash cart and paddles associated with TV hospital dramas. When the crash cart is called for, an electric shock is delivered to a patient's heart during cardiac arrest or if the heart is experiencing arrhythmia. This can reestablish normal contractions (rhythms) in the heart, allowing the patient to survive a life-and-death situation.

The medical term for the procedure is *defibrillation* and now people without formal medical training can be taught to use automated external defibrillators (AEDs), standard equipment today in airports, convention centres and other facilities where large numbers of people congregate. Local chapters of both the Red Cross and (in the US) the American Heart Association teach people how to safely and effectively use AEDs.

In addition, they teach standard cardiopulmonary resuscitation (CPR). CPR has been the mainstay of keeping alive someone who has stopped breathing or whose heart has stopped pumping while you await professional help.

While saving your own life through better eating and being more physically active, you might just want to learn how to save someone else's life in an emergency.

HOW IT WORKS: Repair or replacement of a faulty valve usually requires open-heart surgery. Repair entails restoring the functioning of the existing valve. A surgeon will try to repair your own valve whenever possible. Replacement uses either a *biologic* valve – one obtained from a human cadaver or modified from a pig or cow valve – or an *artificial* valve made from synthetic materials.

BEFORE THE PROCEDURE: Because you will be under general anaesthesia, you will be instructed not to eat or drink for eight to twelve hours before the surgery.

DURING THE PROCEDURE: You will be connected to a heart-lung machine that does the work of those two organs for the duration of the operation; the heart's beating is temporarily stopped while blood flows through the machine instead. The old valve is repaired, or it is removed and the new one is sewn into place.

AFTER THE PROCEDURE: You will spend two to three days in the intensive care unit so heart function can be monitored continuously, then another week or two in a regular patient room. You may notice an occasional 'clicking noise' or sensation in your chest the first days after surgery if an artificial replacement valve (not human, porcine or bovine) is used. This should occur less often with time and go away completely within the first couple of weeks. (If it gets worse, call your doctor.) Bear in mind that it may take months to feel back to yourself, depending on your health before the surgery. Also, note that you will need to take anticoagulant therapy for at least several months – and for the rest of your life if you have a replacement valve that is artificial. And you must always take antibiotics before dental or surgical procedures because of an increased risk for developing an infection of the valve (endocarditis).

Pacemaker

A small, battery-operated electronic device, a pacemaker is inserted under the skin in the chest to help the heart beat regularly and at an appropriate rate. It's commonly used when the natural pacing or conduction system of the heart no longer functions properly. A pacemaker senses when the heart rate is getting too slow or too fast and shifts the rate in the appropriate direction. It also helps the heart to beat more efficiently, adding to pumping capacity in those with weakened heart performance, such as people with congestive heart failure.

HOW IT WORKS: Wires go from a generator through a large vein to the heart, sending electrical impulses that cause the heart to beat. The generator contains the battery as well as the 'information' for regulating the heartbeat and weighs only about 1 ounce. The battery lasts seven to eight years.

BEFORE THE PROCEDURE: Usually you will be told to restrict food and fluid for a period of time before the procedure.

DURING THE PROCEDURE: Inserting a pacemaker takes approximately one hour. You will be awake but given pain medication. A small incision is made in the chest and a small pocket underneath the skin is created. Then, using guidance via X-rays, leads are positioned in the heart, from where they are connected to the generator. Finally, the pacemaker is placed in the pocket and the incision is closed.

AFTER THE PROCEDURE: People who have a pacemaker must carry an identification card – in case they ever lose consciousness. They must also notify people operating certain common devices because those devices – electronic anti-theft surveillance systems, metal detectors, MRI machines and therapeutic radiation apparatus for treating cancer – can throw off the pacemaker's electric signals. (Home appliances carry little to no risk.)

Pacemaker Variation: Internal Defibrillator

Internal defibrillators are sometimes implanted in people who are very vulnerable to life-threatening heart rhythm disturbances. A personalized, micro-mini version of a crash cart and paddles, it jolts the heart whenever necessary.

CARDIAC REHABILITATION:
A KEY TO LONG-TERM RECOVERY

While not technically a procedure, cardiac rehabilitation is the culmination of many procedures that people go through – or the culmination of aggressive treatment they may have received in the wake of a heart attack or other serious cardiovascular problem. Simply put, it is a professionally guided programme to teach women and men heart-healthy lifestyle habits that includes a prescriptive exercise programme once their heart disease has been attended to medically.

It has been estimated that cardiac rehabilitation could prevent the premature deaths of hundreds of thousands of people. But here's the irony:

while the United States is the best place in the world to be if you're in the throes of a heart attack or need intricate surgery to clear a clogged artery (or bypass one that's too far gone), low-tech and low-cost cardiac rehabilitation is underutilized. Only 10 to 20 per cent of those eligible actually end up participating.

Why? In large part, the medical community to date has been more devoted to aggressive treatment of an existing cardiovascular problem than to prevention of further problems down the road. Not enough people are referred.

We believe that approach needs rethinking. Cardiac rehabilitation is a golden opportunity not just to avoid a second heart attack or angioplasty but also to receive what's essentially a personalized health makeover. In the UK the most common form of cardiac rehabilitation is a 6–10 week hospital based programme starting about 4–12 weeks after discharge. Patients take part in an exercise class and a programme of talks covering such topics as heart disease, smoking, stress and diet. There may also be relaxation or stress management classes.

In addition there exists a Heart Manual project with trained facilitators, mainly nurses and health visitors in primary care or community trusts, supported by the NHS. It is in use by 70 health care providers ranging from entire health authority areas to single handed GP practices and is used by about 5,000 patients a year.

The Heart Manual is a six week self-help programme consisting of visits, interviews and health education including relaxation training. It is started as soon as possible after the patient's heart attack. The Heart Manual is proven to be clinically effective, and after a trial, found to be better than hospitatl based rehabilitation at reducing readmission to hospital.

We strongly urge you to lobby for cardiac rehabilitation should you find yourself in the hospital for a serious cardiovascular problem or procedure. In most cases, all you need is your doctor's referral.

Incidentally, Pearl, the woman quoted at the beginning of this chapter, was lucky enough to be referred to cardiac rehabilitation right after her heart attack. Because of it, she never smoked another cigarette – and learned a fair amount about exercise and diet, too.

CHAPTER 11

It's *Your* Turn!

───── ◆ ─────

*If I had known then what I know now, I would have put up much more
of a ruckus than I did.*

— DeLinda

One night in January, DeLinda recounts, 'I woke in the middle of the
night. I just didn't feel right. I was really cold up around my shoulders. I was having trouble breathing. You know when there's just
something not right in your body.'

DeLinda's husband started to drive her to the hospital. But she was feeling so poorly that they stopped at the local fire station. And none too soon.
Her blood pressure had spiked to 225 over 110 and her pulse rate was 44 –
too low for someone who's not an athlete.

The fire department took DeLinda to the emergency room, where the
nightmare she was going through began to take on a new dimension. 'They
gave me some blood pressure medication and referred me to my general
practitioner,' she says. 'They just kind of sloughed me off as having an anxiety attack.'

The next morning, DeLinda phoned her doctor but had to leave a
message. When he called back, she was on the line. The voice mail message he
left was: 'I do not have time to play phone tag'.

Making matters worse still, various medications DeLinda's doctors had
prescribed to lower her blood pressure weren't working well enough. After a
number of feeling-sick, off-hour visits to casualty, she was finally referred to

a cardiologist. The cardiologist put her on a new drug that did help, but for almost two months, DeLinda was too weak to go to work.

It was totally out of character, her daughter, Kim, says. 'My mother's not one to lie around.'

DeLinda then pushed herself to go back to work despite not feeling right (she's the manager of a high-class shoe store) and then one day in mid-March, she began 'feeling really funny in my chest. It wasn't horrible pain. It was more of a burning sensation. I started to go to the hospital. It stopped. I went back to work. I thought, Maybe it's in my head.

'Then the owner of the company came in and said, "You don't look good".' He drove DeLinda to the hospital, where she was told she had bronchitis and prescribed an antibiotic. Her pain at that point was coming in waves. 'One of the nurses thought I had indigestion,' DeLinda recalls. 'I told her I didn't. She asked me, "Do you want to be sick?"'

At eleven o'clock that night, DeLinda sat straight up in bed and said to her husband, 'Andy, I am dying.'

She was doubled over. Andy said he had never seen anyone in so much pain in his life.

He got her to casualty, where she was made to wait for an hour and a half, throwing up and moaning and crying in agony, until she was finally brought to an examining room. An ECG showed she was having a massive heart attack. She was then airlifted to a metropolitan hospital, where she stopped breathing on the table – 'they called Code Blue' and 'paged the chaplain,' Kim says. DeLinda was brought back to life with the crash cart. One of her main coronary arteries was completely blocked.

She is back to work, but only half time. 'She's still a lot more tired than she typically is,' Kim says. 'Before, she was always ready to go do something. Now she has to sit down even in the middle of getting herself dressed. There was a lot of damage done to her heart.'

There is no excuse for what happened to DeLinda (who went on to cardiac rehabilitation). She knew something was wrong, her family knew and even her medical records showed it. This was in 2004, not forty years ago or even ten years ago. Yet no one in a position to help was paying close enough attention. Now, she is paying a very high price. Indeed, at 61, she almost paid the ultimate price.

You never know what your particular circumstances are going to be, but we believe it's possible to help keep things from getting so far out of hand – through advocacy. To get the best out of the health care system, it's crucial that you take an active role and advocate for yourself. DeLinda, with 20/20 hindsight, wholeheartedly agrees. 'I should have gone to the doctor sooner in the first place,' she says. 'I waited too long. It was the holidays. I told myself, "It'll go away."' She also feels she didn't trust her own instincts enough to speak up when she needed to. 'What women have to do is listen to their bodies,' she notes. 'I was taking them at their word. I would definitely speak to the doctors differently if this happened now. I would stay in the doctor's office until I got answers to my questions.'

A lot of women are not comfortable being vocal self-advocates. Women are brought up to be accommodating, respectful, never questioning the status quo or rocking the boat. Women are typically conflict avoiders. But you cannot live a respectful life without first respecting *yourself* to make sure you get the best care possible. Indeed, if you don't treat yourself respectfully, it can *cost* you your life.

It takes courage to advocate for yourself, especially if you're not used to it. But *there are no boundaries to what you can do for yourself if you speak up for your own cause.* It doesn't mean that you have to be rude, but it does mean holding firm. You don't have to take your care or your situation at face value. DeLinda was in no way responsible for the poor and sometimes callous medical treatment she received, but if she had known how to work the system better, perhaps she would have got the help she needed months earlier and avoided a lot of heart muscle damage.

That's what this chapter is about: working the system through advocating for yourself. You need to find the fortitude for that within your own mind; with friends and family; with your doctor and other health care professionals; and, if necessary, at the hospital.

HOW YOU TALK TO YOURSELF

The most important discussion you're ever going to have about your heart health is the one you have with yourself. For better or worse, *you* are the one who's ultimately responsible for your own primary care. Everything else flows from that. Of course, if you're reading this book, you've already been having that most important internal dialogue and taking the reins to be more aware of your own health. By learning what you can do for yourself lifestyle-wise to protect your heart and also by learning a lot of the technical terminology related to heart health and heart disease, you have put yourself in a better position to have meaningful interactions with your health care providers – doctors, nurses and so on.

But you also need a plan to put your knowledge into action; change doesn't come easily. Even something as simple as making sure to eat at least seven servings of vegetables and fruit a day is not an easy task if you've spent decades following a different kind of eating pattern. You also need to plan regular doctor's visits; that's a crucial part of living a healthy lifestyle.

It's simple enough to make a plan. You write it down so you can check off what you've accomplished as you go along. It's how you talk to yourself about your plan – how you do or do not advocate for yourself – that can get in the way.

Psychologists talk about it in terms of triggers. There are five types of triggers: cognitive, emotional, environmental, physical and social. They can be positive or negative, depending on whether they enhance your ability to do something for yourself or interfere.

For instance, a negative *cognitive* trigger, which is a trigger based on how you think about your predicament, would be: 'I don't have time to exercise'. That might seem irrefutable – after all, most women lead busy lives. But a way around it might be to actually sit down with a calendar or day planner and see where it would be possible to wedge in exercise. Perhaps it comes down to missing a certain television show a few nights a week, getting up a little earlier several times a week, getting a neighbour to watch the kids for an hour here or there, or joining a gym on your commuting route. Whatever the answer, 'I don't have time to exercise' becomes a different tape playing in your head because you no longer accept it as a given and actively look for ways to work exercise into what is probably an already packed schedule.

A negative *emotional* trigger might be guilt – which is very common in people who want to make a change but don't. The guilt ends up sucking up all the emotional energy that should be going towards the change, when it would be better for a woman to tell herself that even a small change, such as eating another vegetable every day or using the stairs for three flights, is a start. It's amazing how one small step leads to another until there's significant momentum and the guilt is very effectively replaced with actions that, before long, turn into habits.

It's the same for *environmental, physical* and *social* triggers. If your home environment is such that caloric treats high in saturated or *trans* fat are always around instead of fruit and low-fat yogurt, *of course* your environment is going to work against you. If, on the other hand, you feel like having cake, sweets or ice cream but the only options in the house are plain non-fat yogurt topped with berries or already-cut watermelon chunks and pineapple rings, your environment can't sabotage your efforts. (If it's not a black-and-white issue because others in the household are not as committed as you are to following a heart-healthy diet, you may have to set up 'safe zones' in the cupboards or refrigerator shelves to minimize temptation. The degree to which such artificial barriers can help is amazing. They keep your priorities in the front of your mind.)

If *physically* speaking, you always feel too tired to take care of yourself by exercising, you need to remind yourself that while anticipating making changes to your exercise pattern can seem exhausting and may even feel very tiring at first, people who get some physical activity most days of the week and also eat right report feeling heightened energy after just a short time. Similarly, making the necessary dietary changes may seem like work at the beginning – you have to get used to grocery shopping and preparing food regularly – but once they become the 'default' mode, they are no more time-consuming than the habits you currently have.

Finally, if your *social* triggers are holding you back – your friends would rather sit around over a mocha latte rather than take a walk – it's important not to let them stand in your way. (More on that shortly.)

It's all about finding your *inner strength*. You need to advocate for yourself when another part of you is whispering undermining messages in your ear. It's crucial, because it not only lets you live more healthily, it also lets you speak up for yourself to others when you need to. When you are strong you'll never let the inclination to be polite stand in the way of your health.

To help you become your own best advocate, to be assertive about taking care of yourself properly, here are some questions to ask yourself. They sound simple on the surface but get to the root of tackling the problem.

- When was the last time I went to the doctor for a thorough physical? (If it has been longer than two years, make an appointment now.)
- When am I going to get to the shop to buy some new athletic shoes?
- When am I going to exercise this week? Which days work for me? What time of day can I fit it in? (By all means get out your calendar or diary and write it down. Don't just go through it in your head.)
- What errands can I do this week by walking instead of driving?
- What strategy can I use to ensure that I follow my 'kitchen closed' policy after dinner? How will I handle it if someone else in the house has a snack after I'm done eating for the evening? With what will I replace eating while watching television?
- How can I buy the most wholesome take-out dinners on evenings that I know I won't have time to cook? How will I ensure appropriate portion control once I get those meals home? Will I put half in the refrigerator before I sit down to eat? Will I dole out a portion that's supposedly meant for one person to two or even three people in the household?
- At what time of day can I take twenty minutes to just sit and relax, read my book or meditate?

HOW YOU TALK TO OTHERS IN YOUR CIRCLE

Once you've embraced the idea that you're going to be your own best advocate, it's important to let others know where you stand – and bring them on board, if possible. In the best of all possible worlds, your spouse or others with whom you are close are totally with you, happy to go along with changes you want to make to the meals and snacks that come out of the kitchen along with scheduling changes to accommodate your exercise regimen.

But a lot of spouses and others close to you may simply stay out of it. You have to make decisions for yourself, even if your husband, partner, children or friends don't want to go along. That doesn't mean you have a bad marriage or family life or even unsupportive significant others. But it probably does mean that you'll have to do things a little differently from others in your life – and not backtrack because you don't want to seem like a spoilsport. After all, if your loved ones have a right to their lifestyle habits without running them by you first, you have a right to yours.

By the same token, your family and friends are entitled to their latte, if they want it. You need to be clear with them that you are committed to your lifestyle changes and that they have to respect you enough to support you in your efforts, even if they don't want to join in. But you don't need to start preaching. In fact, you can even order a coffee with skimmed milk during the latte fests so as not to lose out on good socializing. A woman can work within *any* situation if she prepares ahead of time.

Sometimes, your new resolve may even interest some otherwise uninterested parties in making heart-healthy changes themselves. Whether or not that happens, it pays to work at actively identifying other people in your life who might be good candidates for becoming more directly involved in helping you meet your heart-health goals – or who at least will not try to hold you back from doing what you need to do because it changes the status quo. It's easier if you don't have to go it totally alone.

The most obvious and natural pool of people outside your home are your friends, colleagues or other family members you count among your friends – siblings, grown children and so on. Maybe they'll want to exercise with you, or share recipes with you, or just be willing to engage in a running dialogue with you about the strides you're making and the hurdles you have to cross.

Like-minded people can come from a broader circle, too. It's easier than you think. Maybe you'll start talking to a neighbour you frequently see on her daily walk. Or perhaps you'll find someone who walks regularly at work during lunchtime and ask if you can join her.

Sometimes you may want to *hire* players for your 'support group'. Maybe it's a good time to make an appointment with a psychotherapist who can help you work through some old issues that have kept you from moving ahead. Maybe paying for several sessions with a personal trainer to help you get the hang of strength training is what you need to jump-start your exercise efforts.

Whether the person or people are part of your social network or professionals you pay for their expertise, enlisting others in your cause is one of the best ways to take care of yourself and make sure you're *getting taken care of* at the same time.

Indeed, having people in your corner can enhance your actual medical care. DeLinda's daughter, Kim, for instance, remembers that her mother 'started feeling extremely tired and short of breath' earlier than she herself remembers – important information for medical professionals in their assessment and treatment. She knew, too, that the problem must be her mother's heart even when others were not identifying it. 'I'm no doctor,' Kim says. 'But you go to a reputable site on the Internet. You do a little research. You put two and two together.' In other words, having someone on your team can encourage you to keep seeking treatment even when you and others around you have doubts.

Kim only wishes, in fact, that she had advocated *more* strongly for her mother – and certainly wouldn't hesitate to do so in the future. Having been there for some of the visits to casualty, she says that if she could do it over again, 'I would have kept asking, "What is causing all this pain and discomfort?" I would have pressed more. I felt this incredible sense of frustration.

'My brother's wife is a nurse. She told me, "You're going to have to ask questions and keep asking and push and push and push."' Now Kim knows just how true those words of advice were.

Following are some things you might say to those in your inner circle to make sure you get what you need from them:

- *To a friend:* I am starting a walking programme and can't think of someone I'd rather walk with than you. Would you consider making a commitment to walk with me for a half hour just twice a week? I don't mean a stroll; I really need to *walk*. But we can still talk and connect during that time.
- *To a husband and children:* I need you to stop making fun of my new choices. I'm not telling you that you can't snack on whatever you'd like. But I deserve the same respect. If you can't be on my side in this, at least don't try to sabotage my efforts.
- *To colleagues:* I know I've never ordered this way before when we've gone out to lunch. But I'm really trying to make an effort to eat better for heart health. Please don't give me a hard time. I need your support right now.
- *To kids:* If you see the bedroom door closed, unless it is an emergency, please wait twenty minutes. I need that uninterrupted time to unwind.

- *To family:* I would like to take a vacation this year that allows me to be more active with hiking and bicycling. But I know you guys love to loll on the beach. Let's choose a place that will meet all our wishes.
- *To a yoga instructor:* I have high cholesterol and am really stressed out. What can you tell me about your class? What are the other participants like? I'm beginning an exercise programme, but are they all starting out fitter than I am? I need to push myself, but I have to be comfortable enough to be able to stick with it – and enjoy it.

HOW YOU TALK TO YOUR DOCTOR

Despite her regrets about not speaking up more for herself during her medical nightmare, there is one way DeLinda took care of herself that she is very pleased with. She signed on with a new general practitioner after it was clear her doctor was not the one for her. Once the two of them did finally speak about her symptoms after the 'phone tag' incident, DeLinda says that 'he treated me like, "Get over it." I never went back.'

It was actually her new doctor who referred her to a cardiologist. The medication he had prescribed was not bringing down her blood pressure adequately and he told her point-blank, 'I'm not trained to deal with what's going on'.

DeLinda is very glad about having made the decision to change doctors. But there's more to getting the most out of your medical team than respecting yourself enough not to accept anything less than respect from others. And there's more than asking the right questions and not backing down during a crisis. There's also advocating for yourself by talking with your doctor and asking the right questions *all along.*

Imagine if your doctor told you that you had high cholesterol and wanted to see you in six weeks to retest it – and said that if your cholesterol didn't come down, she or he was going to prescribe statin drugs. Then, imagine if you walked in after six weeks and said, 'I've lost five pounds, I'm walking almost every day and I'm eating more fruits and vegetables and fewer heavy desserts. If my cholesterol is coming down but still is not low enough, what else can I do?'

A lot will have changed in your relationship with your health care provider. One thing is that most assuredly your doctor will listen to you and be much more willing to work *with* you rather than 'from above'. Perhaps even more important, *you'll* feel emboldened – and less flustered by the prospect of being in the doctor's office. You'll also expect more from your doctor because you will have expected more from yourself. You'll be more inclined to ask yourself, either consciously or unconsciously, 'Is my doctor up to the mark?'

It's important to write down your questions before going to the doctor's office so you don't end up forgetting something that's important to you. In this day of managed care, doctors are under tremendous time constraints and the better prepared you are, the better use you'll be able to make of what might be a short visit. The two of us are strong women who have no problem speaking up for ourselves when we see our doctors, but still, each of us writes down a list of questions to ask so that we get the most out of our visits. For many, it also cuts down on nervousness.

Some questions you might want to ask your health care provider:

- *What are my numbers?* Everyone should be aware of her blood lipids (cholesterol and triglycerides) and blood pressure. Even if they're in the desirable range, you want to know if they're going up. You want to be able to assess risk for yourself. By the same token, you want to know if your lifestyle measures are working and the numbers are going down – and to what degree. Ask for a copy of your reports.
- *Can I get sessions with a dietitian?* If your cholesterol, triglycerides, blood pressure or glucose is high and you're overweight or simply aware that you need to follow a more healthful diet but don't know how, counselling with a registered dietitian can help bring your numbers into line – often without drugs. If you have health insurance, many companies pay for the sessions with a referral from your doctor.
- *Are there diagnostic tests I should be getting to make sure we know the root of the problem?* (For instance, as we explained in chapter 9, high LDL-cholesterol is sometimes a sign of a thyroid problem rather than a cardiovascular problem, meaning a simple blood test might be in order.)

- *Should I also be seeing a cardiologist?* (Cardiologists generally don't treat high LDL-cholesterol or high blood pressure, but there are always exceptions, as DeLinda's story shows.)
- *What are the potential side effects of the medications you're prescribing?* How should I take the drugs? With food? Between meals? At a certain time of day? What should I do if I miss a dose or run out of pills and have forgotten to get a repeat prescription?
- *When can I expect to see results with my new treatment?* If I am compliant with the medications and I exercise more, lose weight and eat better, what degree of improvement can I expect?
- *What symptoms should prompt me to see you again before the next scheduled appointment?* (You should also bring up any symptoms you have been having that are out of the ordinary. Maybe you're getting winded more easily doing household chores like changing the sheets or carrying a bag of groceries. Doctors can work with specifics like these to get to a diagnosis – and appropriate treatment – faster.)
- *Is there anyone else in your office I can communicate with if I have questions and you're not available?* A nurse? A medical partner?
- *Is it best to reach you directly by leaving a message with your receptionist or by e-mailing you?*

Good doctors who will answer your questions and re-answer them if you don't understand their explanations the first time around, come in both sexes and all ages. What's central is their attitude towards *you*. If you're not comfortable with your doctor or feel she or he gives you short shrift, switch.

HOW YOU TALK TO HEALTH PROFESSIONALS IN CASUALTY

In the unlikely event that you end up going to casualty for heart-related symptoms, there are a number of things you need to know so that you can advocate for yourself most effectively. One is not to delay. We can't stress this enough. If you think, for instance, that there's even a remote chance you are having a heart attack or stroke, don't wait to see whether it passes. And don't tell yourself it's nothing. Many women make the dangerous mistake of minimizing

You May Be More Capable Than You're Told

If you have an unstable condition that puts your health at immediate risk, it's very important to do what your doctor says to get things under control. But if it's a condition that is stable and has been going on for a long time, there's a chance you're more capable of living normally than you may be told.

We have heard a number of stories from people who have gone to see a doctor for their hearts and were cautioned not even to break a sweat or lift more than 5 pounds. One active person we know – a jogger and tennis player as well as avid gardener – had a congenital heart murmur that wasn't diagnosed until an annual physical at age 40. Her doctor referred her to a cardiologist, who had a cardiology resident examine her via an echocardiogram before coming into the room to follow up. The young resident told her that she was not allowed to lift any weight heavier than 10 pounds and that running was out of the question.

The woman was devastated – her whole life was going to be turned upside down. Fortunately, she brought it up with the cardiologist when he came in to examine her. He told her such advice was unwarranted. She might need a valve replacement many years down the line, he said, but even that was unlikely. If she hadn't spoken up and gotten her 'second opinion', she would have walked around on tiptoes – unnecessarily – and suffered a *decline* in her heart health from lack of activity.

what they're going through. This could be a matter of life and death. Delaying can also increase the amount of permanent damage that occurs. *Don't minimize.* Get someone to drive you to the hospital – immediately. If no one's available, call 999.

Once at the hospital, tell the triage nurse you suspect it's a heart attack or some other heart-related problem. Don't feel funny about it and don't let anyone tell you it's not possible because you're a woman or because your symptoms are not typical of a heart attack. Remember, women's heart attack symptoms are often diffuse. A heart attack could feel more like indigestion than a train running over your chest. If you have another person with you, so much the better. He or she can fill in where you might not be able to because of pain or anxiety about what's going on.

OUR CHARGE TO YOU

Taking the reins and becoming your own advocate, which in turn makes *others* your advocates, may not be easy. Nor is it easy to change eating and exercise habits that may have been ingrained for decades. But you are at a place in your life where you need to make a decision. You need to weigh whether you are willing to make the necessary changes to improve your heart health and perhaps even extend your life.

We know you can do it. In the two decades that we have been talking to women about their bodies, we have seen that strong women come in all shapes, ages, sizes and mind-sets. No matter what their starting point, they have been able to make fundamental shifts in how they live their lives. And the rewards are so worth the effort, as many of the women we spoke with confirmed.

Anne, who was able to take lifestyle steps to lower her cholesterol, says that she could do it because she took charge of her own situation. It was *she* who made sure her doctor finally sent a sample of her blood to a lab for cholesterol analysis. It was also she who got her doctor to pay closer attention to her blood pressure. Because it hadn't quite reached the threshold for 'high,' her doctor kept telling her not to worry about it. But she kept asking him, 'Don't you think it's high for *me*, since I live such a healthy lifestyle?' It was then that closer tabs began to be kept and they could catch it when it went above 140/90.

Deanne, the woman who improved her heart health by losing weight, says that her best advice 'is simply to keep reminding yourself that you can do whatever you want to.' A lot of women feel defeated before they even begin, she remarks, but 'don't let anyone stand in your way; have confidence in yourself.' The payback for that attitude and approach: 'I wake up every day and have this incredible feeling of being healthy and happy,' Deanne says.

Wendy, who also changed her eating style to keep down her cholesterol, expresses it more bluntly. When you do things right for yourself, she says, 'you don't feel 'bad' anymore. You're doing every part of your body, not just your heart, a good favour. The minute I started taking care of my body, I knew that. I know a lot of women think it's hopeless. But it's not. Rant and rave if you have to. Moan about how difficult it is. But then do something about it. You've got to start right now.'

We agree. Your life really depends on making the changes. Better still, you will likely enjoy collateral benefits. Women are frequently at the centre of their circle of family and friends. How we live our lives often directly impacts how others we care about live theirs. Furthermore, as you make these fundamental changes, you won't feel deprived. Rather, you'll feel enriched because everything you do for yourself you'll be able to do in a way that works within your own lifestyle. The steps are always flexible enough so that you can find a way to adapt them to your needs and tastes.

As you make the shift, which we believe you are doing even by finishing this book, we wish you health and vitality for years to come. We wish you control over your own life. And we wish you a strong heart. From this point forward, it will become stronger still.

Glossary

Aerobic exercise: Continuous exercise that works the entire cardiovascular system, including the heart and lungs, by elevating the heart rate. Examples include brisk walking, running, bicycling and swimming.

Alpha-linolenic acid (ALA): A type of omega-3 fatty acid found in certain plant foods and plant oils, such as rapeseed and soya bean oils, walnuts and flaxseeds. Only a small amount of ALA can be converted to the type of omega-3s found in fish.

Aneurysm: The abnormal enlargement or bulging of a section of an artery caused by damage to or weakness in the vessel wall. Aneurysms can occur in any type of blood vessel, but they almost always form in an artery.

Angina (an-JI-nuh): Chest pain or discomfort that occurs when the heart muscle does not get enough oxygenated blood. It may feel like pressure or a squeezing pain in your chest. The pain may also be felt in the shoulders, arms, neck, jaw or back. Sometimes it feels like indigestion.

Angioplasty (AN jee oh-plas-tee): A medical procedure used to open narrowed or clogged blood vessels of the heart.

Antioxidant: A nutrient or chemical that can 'absorb' or block damage caused by substances known as free radicals, thereby protecting body tissue.

Arrhythmia: Refers to any change from the normal sequence of electrical impulses in the heart, causing abnormal heart rhythms.

Arteries: Blood vessels that carry oxygen-rich blood from the heart to all the cells in the body.

Atherosclerosis (ath-er-o-skle-RO-sis): The hardening and narrowing of the arteries caused by the slow buildup of plaque on the inside of the artery walls.

Atrial fibrillation: The heart's two small upper chambers – the left and right atria – quiver instead of beating effectively. Blood isn't pumped completely out of them, so it may pool and clot. If a piece of a blood clot in the atria leaves the heart and becomes lodged in an artery in the brain, a stroke results. About 15 per cent of strokes occur in people with atrial fibrillation.

Atrium (right and left) (AY-tree-um): The atria (plural of 'atrium') are the two upper chambers of the heart that collect blood as it flows in.

Bicuspid valve: Also known as the mitral (MI-trul) valve, the bicuspid valve is located on the left side of the heart, between the left atrium and the left ventricle.

Blood pressure (systolic and diastolic): The force of the blood pushing against the walls of the arteries as it's pumped out of the heart with each beat. Blood pressure is at its highest when the heart beats, pumping the blood. This is called *systolic pressure*. When the heart is at rest, between beats, your blood pressure falls. This is *diastolic pressure*.

Blood vessels: 'Tubes' that carry blood throughout the body. The two main types of blood vessels are arteries and veins. Arteries carry blood *away* from the heart. Veins carry blood back *to* the heart.

Body mass index (BMI): A measure of weight for height. To find your BMI, refer to page 146.

Capillaries: Very small blood vessels that connect arteries to veins. From capillaries, oxygen and nutrients are dropped off by the blood to individual cells. Carbon dioxide and other waste are picked up.

Cardiac catheterization: A catheter, or thin tube, is threaded into the heart, providing information on blood pressure within the heart, how much oxygen is in the blood flowing through the heart and the pumping ability of the heart.

Cardiovascular system: The entire circulatory system of the body, blood vessels, lungs and heart.

Carotid artery stenosis (kah-ROT-id AR-ter-ee sten-O-sis): Narrowing of the carotid arteries, the main arteries in the neck that supply blood to the brain. This is a major risk factor for ischemic (is-KEEM-ik) stroke, the most common form of stroke.

Cholesterol: A waxy substance made by the liver and also supplied in the diet through animal foods such as eggs, meats and dairy products. Cholesterol is needed in the body to insulate nerves, make cell membranes and produce certain hormones. However, the body can make adequate cholesterol, so dietary cholesterol isn't needed. Dietary cholesterol can raise blood cholesterol, but not nearly as much as saturated fat and *trans*-fatty acids.

Congestive heart failure: A condition wherein the heart cannot efficiently pump blood throughout the body. Excess fluid backs up into the lungs, heart and other tissues. The fluid collects, causing congestion.

Coronary artery disease (CAD): Occurs when the arteries that supply blood to the heart muscle (coronary arteries) become narrowed or clogged. Blood flow to the heart becomes compromised, decreasing the oxygen supply to the heart muscle.

Docosohexanoic acid (DHA): An omega-3 fatty acid, found in highest concentrations in cold-water fish. Intakes have been related to decreased risk of heart disease.

Eicosapentaenoic acid (EPA): An omega-3 fatty acid, found in highest concentrations in cold-water fish. Intakes have been related to a reduced risk of heart disease.

Fatty acid: A chain of carbons attached to one another with either single or double bonds. A fatty acid with no double bonds is saturated; a chain with a single double bond is monounsaturated; and a chain with two or more double bonds is polyunsaturated. A *trans*-fatty acid contains one or more double bonds in a less common configuration.

Heart attack (myocardial infarction): Occurs when the supply of blood and oxygen to an area of heart muscle is blocked, usually by a clot in a coronary artery. If the blockage is not treated within minutes to hours, the affected heart muscle will die and be replaced by scar. **A heart attack is an emergency. Call 999 if you think you (or someone else) may be having a heart attack. Prompt treatment of a heart attack can help prevent or limit lasting damage to the heart and can also prevent death.**

Heart contractions: Heart muscle squeezing in rhythmic manner to push blood out of the heart. With each contraction, about 50 per cent of the blood in the heart is pushed out into the body; less in those with congestive heart failure.

Haemorrhagic stroke: The bursting of an artery in the brain, causing bleeding into the brain.

Inflammation: The process by which the body responds to injury. Laboratory evidence and findings from clinical and population studies suggest that inflammation is part of atherosclerosis, the buildup of fatty deposits in artery linings.

Ischemic stroke: Occurs when a clot blocks blood flow in an artery that brings blood to the brain. Accounts for up to 80 per cent of all strokes.

Lipoproteins: These are fat-protein combinations. Because oil (fat) and water (in the blood) don't mix, the fat that circulates in the bloodstream needs to be packaged with protein (and other substances) so it can be transported. The exact makeup of the package determines its role. The three main lipoproteins:

Very Low Density Lipoprotein (VLDL): The major fat-carrying particle in the bloodstream. Delivers fatty acids to all cells in the body for use as energy or storage.

Low Density Lipoprotein (LDL): Commonly referred to as 'bad' LDL, it carries most of the cholesterol in the blood, delivering it

to cells throughout the body. When LDL delivers excess cholesterol to cells in the walls of blood vessels, atherosclerotic plaque
forms.

High Density Lipoprotein (HDL): Commonly referred to as 'good'
HDL, it's the only lipoprotein particle that carries cholesterol
from various cells in the body to the liver for metabolism or ex-
cretion.

Mitral valve (See bicuspid valve.)

Murmur: An unusual, or extra, sound heard during your heartbeat. In
adults, murmurs are most often due to heart valve problems that cause a
little blood to flow backward rather than forward.

Myocardial infarction (See heart attack.)

Omega-3 fatty acids: A family of fatty acids that is essential to human health,
found in relatively large quantities in cold-water fish. Also found in certain plant foods and plant oils, such as rapeseed and soya bean oils, walnuts and flaxseeds. Plant-based omega-3s are not as heart-protective.
(See also DHA and EPA.)

Peripheral vascular disease: Peripheral vascular disease (PVD) is atherosclerosis of blood vessels other than those of the heart or brain. It predominantly involves the vasculature of the legs or arms. The most common
and important type of PVD is peripheral arterial disease, or PAD, which
affects 8 to 12 million Americans. It becomes more common as one gets
older and by age 70, about 20 per cent of the population is affected. Diagnosis is critical, as people with PAD face a six to seven times higher risk
of heart attack or stroke.

Plaque: Made up primarily of cholesterol and sometimes calcium, it can
build up inside an artery where, in time, it may restrict blood flow.

Recommended Daily Allowance (RDA): The reference numbers developed
by the government that are used for food labelling. The % RDA for a

nutrient gives a general idea of a food's contribution of that nutrient to the total daily diet.

Stent: A tiny mesh tube. It is inserted during angioplasty to keep open a narrowed artery. Some stents are coated with medication to help prevent the artery from closing again.

Strength training (progressive resistance training): A mode of exercise in which the muscles work against enough resistance to challenge them and thereby increase strength. An example is weight lifting.

Stroke (See haemorrhagic stroke and ischemic stroke.)

Transient ischemic attack (TIA): A 'mini-stroke' that produces strokelike symptoms but no lasting damage. TIAs occur when a blood clot temporarily clogs an artery and part of the brain doesn't get the blood it needs. Symptoms occur rapidly and generally last about one minute.

Tricuspid (tri-CUSS-pid) **valve:** On the right side of the heart, located between the right atrium and the right ventricle.

Triglycerides: The form of fat found in foods and body fat cells. Triglycerides are used for energy or storage.

Veins: Blood vessels that carry blood back to the heart after it has dropped off oxygen and nutrients throughout the body and picked up waste material, including carbon dioxide.

Ventricles (VEN-trih-kuls): The two lower chambers of the heart that pump blood out of the heart to the lungs or other parts of the body.

Weight-bearing exercise: Aerobic exercises that require the legs to support the weight of the body. Walking is weight bearing. Swimming and biking are not.

Resources

◆

We list here numerous resources for more information about heart health and related issues. The list includes organizations, books, websites and more. Please bear in mind that websites frequently change. The sites listed here were accessible when we compiled this section. If any one of them is inoperative at a later date, we encourage you to use a reliable search engine to locate the source at its new site.

General Heart Health Resources

The British Heart Foundation is the leading national charity fighting heart disease:

British Heart Foundation
14 Fitzhardinge Street
London W1H 6DH
020 7935 0185
Heart Information Line 08450 708070
www.bhf.org.uk
www.bhfactive.org.uk (for information on physical activity)

The Department of Health has a website at www.dh.gov.uk
For specific information, search for coronary heart disease.

There is more Department of Health information on
www.prodigy.nhs.uk/ClinicalGuidance

The National Health Service website is www.nhsdirect.nhs.uk

The Stroke Association is the only national charity solely concered with
combating stroke in people of all ages, and helps stroke patients directly
through its community services. Their website is www.stroke.org.uk

For information on The Red Dress Campaign specifically aimed at women,
go to the website of the Cardiothoracic Centre at Liverpool NHS Trust. Web
address: www.ctc.nhs.uk/heartdisease

Useful information on heart health is also available at www.netdoctor.co.uk
and specific information about support groups at can be found at their web
page www.netdoctor.co.uk/directory/support_groups

Books on Heart Disease and Related Topics

The following books include heart-healthy recipes:

The Light-Hearted Cookbook, recipes for a healthy heart, by Anne Lindsay,
    Grub Street, 1999. Published with the British Heart Foundation.

The Everyday Light-Hearted Cookbook, by Anne Lindsay, Grub Street, 1994.
    Published with the British Heart Foundation.

The Everyday Low-Fat Cookbook, Anne Lindsay, Grub Street, 2003.

*Women Are Not Small Men: Life-Saving Strategies for Preventing and Healing
    Heart Disease in Women,* Neica Goldberg, MD, Ballantine Books, 2003.

The Female Heart: The Truth About Women and Heart Disease, Marianne
    Legato, MD and Carol Colman, Quill, 2000.

Dr Susan Love's Menopause and Hormone Book: Making Informed Choices,
    Susan M. Love, MD and Karen Lindsay, Times Books, 1998.

Giving up Smoking

The British Heart Foundation has a website with specific information on smoking: www.bhf.org.uk/smoking

The National Health service advice and information can be found at www.givingupsmoking.co.uk

QUIT is the national charity helping people give up smoking. Their website is www.quit.org.uk

There is a BUPA health factsheet at www.bupa.co.uk:80/health_information/asp/healthy_living/lifestyle/smoking

More information is available on www.netdoctor.co.uk/smoking and on the Department of Health website www.dh.gov.uk/policyandguidance/health-andsocialcaretopics/tobacco

Dr Nelson's Website and Books

www.strongwomen.com has a free electronic newsletter and animated exercise programmes as well as other useful information regarding nutrition and exercise.

Strong Women Stay Young, Miriam E. Nelson, PhD, with Sarah Wernick, PhD, Aurum Press Ltd, 2000.

Strong Women Stay Slim, Miriam E. Nelson, PhD, with Sarah Wernick, PhD, Aurum Press Ltd, 1999.

Strong Women, Strong Bones, Miriam E. Nelson, PhD, with Sarah Wernick, PhD, Piatkus Books, 2000.

Strong Women Eat Well, Miriam E. Nelson, PhD, with Judy Knipe, Lothian Books, 2001.

Strong Women and Men *Beat Arthritis,* Miriam E. Nelson, PhD, Kristin Baker, PhD and Ronenn Roubenoff, MD, MSH, with Lawrence Lindner, MA, Aurum Press Ltd, 2003.

The Strong Women's Journal, Miriam E. Nelson, PhD, Perigee, 2003.

Tufts University Resources

The John Hancock Center for Physical Activity and Nutrition at the Friedman School of Nutrition Science and Policy, Tufts University, maintains a website with useful information regarding ongoing programmes such as the community-based StrongWomen Program: www.go.tufts.edu/JHCPAN

The Tufts University Health & Nutrition Letter, an eight-page monthly newsletter, has been called 'the best available source of news and views on nutrition' by *US News & World Report* and has also received accolades from *The New York Times, The Boston Globe and* the *Columbia Journalism Review,* among other publications. Go to: www.healthletter.tufts.edu

Organizations

The following organizations supply comprehensive information about nutrition, physical activity and numerous other health-related topics.

General Medical Council holds the register of all doctors qualified to practise in the UK
www.gmc-uk.org

The National Health Service's website is at www.nhsdirect.nhs.uk

The Health Professions Council regulates dietitians, physiotherapists etc.
www.hpc-uk.org

Committee on Safety of Medicines
www.mca.gov.uk

Food Standards Agency
www.foodstandards.gov.uk

Doctor Patient Partnerships
www.dpp.org.uk

The Chartered Society of Physiotherapy is the profession body for the UK's chartered physiotherapists. It has links with other groups which cater for different specialities.

www.csp.org.uk

To find a chartered physiotherapist near you

www.physio2u.org.uk

The British Dietetic Association (BDA) is the professional association of state registered dietitians.

0121 200 8080

www.bda.uk.com

The Register of Exercise Professionals (REPs)

Charter House

29A London Road

Croydon, Surrey CR0 2RE

www.reps-uk.org

The British Association of Sports Exercise Medicine (BASEM) certifies fitness professionals

www.basem.co.uk

The British Association of Sport and Exercise Sciences (BASES) has a website with accredited consultants.

www.bases.org.uk

The British Cardiac Society for information on cardiac rehabilitation and other topics

www.bcs.com

A website developed by the University of York with information for patients

www.cardiacrehabilitation.org.uk

For information on Trascendental Meditation go to www.t-m.org.uk or www.tm-london.org.uk

Institute of Complementary Medicine
www.i-c-m.org.uk

The British Wheel of Yoga
01529 306851
www.bwy.org.uk

The Tai Chi Union for Great Britian for a list of recognized classes in your area:
0141 810 3482
www.taichiunion.com

Books and Other Resources with Reliable Nutrition, Exercise and Weight Control Information

The American Dietetic Association's Complete Food & Nutrition Guide, Roberta Larson Duyff, MS, RD, John Wiley & Sons Inc, 2002.

The Step Diet Book, James Hill, PhD, John Peters, PhD, with Bonnie Jortberg, MS, RD, Workman Publishing, 2004.

The Complete Guide to Walking for Health, Weight Loss and Fitness, Mark Fenton, The Lyons Press, 2001.

The Spark: A Revolutionary New Plan to Get Fit and Lose Weight, Glenn A. Gaesser, PhD and Karla Dougherty, Simon & Schuster, 2001.

Thin for Life: 10 Keys to Success from People Who Have Lost Weight and Kept It Off, Anne Fletcher, MS, R., Houghton Mifflin Company, 2003.

Exercise Equipment

For pedometers try local sports equipment shops or the following websites.

Quality pedometers UK at www.polygondirect.com

Pedometers at Amazon at Amazon.co.uk/personalcare

Silva pedometers UK at www.ukge.co.uk

Pedometers co uk at www.pedometers.co.uk

Totally fitness at www.totallyfitness.co.uk

BodyPower Sports plc
Unit 7, Carousel Way
Riverside Business Park
Northampton NN3 9HG
01604 773220
www.bodypower.co.uk

Fitness Peak
16-20 Regent Street
Leeds LS2 7OA
0113 244 2242
0800 028 2684
www.fitnesspeak.co.uk

Physical Company Ltd
2a Desborough Industrial Park
Desborough Park Road
High Wycombe, Bucks HP12 3BG
014994 769222
www.physicalcompany.co.uk

Powerhouse Fitness
Unit 11, 12 Whitehall Street
Glasgow C3 8BN
0141 221 3885
0800 221 3885

www.powerhouse-fitness.co.uk

Premier Sports and Fitness
9-11 Darlington Street
Wigan WN1 1DL
01942 495695
www.premiersportsandfitness.co.uk

ProActive Health Ltd   (stocks US ankle weights)
Quarry Court, Bell Lane
Cassington, Oxon OX29 4DS
01865 886300
and
18 Coombend Road
Radstock
Bath, Avon BA3 3AT
01761 439900
www.proactive-health.co.uk

Totally Fitness
108 Crawford Street
London W1H 2JB
020 7467 5925
www.totallyfitness.com
www.totallyfitness.co.uk

Bibliography

◆

General Heart Disease

Chobanian, A. V., Bakris, G. L., Black, H. R. , Cushman, W. C. , et al. National High Blood Pressure Education Program Coordinating Committee. Seventh Report of the Joint National Committee on Prevention, Detection, Evaluation and Treatment of High Blood Pressure. *Hypertension.* 2003; 42: 1206–52.

Expert Panel on Detection, Evaluation and Treatment of High Blood Cholesterol in Adults. Executive summary of the Third Report of the National Cholesterol Education Program (NCEP) Expert Panel on Detection, Evaluation and Treatment of High Blood Cholesterol in Adults (Adult Treatment Panel III). *Journal of the American Medical Association.* 2001; 285: 2486–97.

Grundy, S. M., Cleeman, J. I., Merz, C.N., Brewer, B., et al., for the Coordinating Committee of the National Cholesterol Education Program. Implications of Recent Clinical Trials for the National Cholesterol Education Program. Adult Treatment Panel III Guidelines. *Circulation.* 2004; 110: 227–39.

Krauss, R. M., Eckel, R. H., Howard, B., Appel, L. J., et al. American Heart Association Dietary Guidelines: revision 2000: A Statement for Healthcare Professionals from the Nutrition Committee of the American Heart Association. *Circulation* 2002; 102: 2284–99.

Pearson, T. A., Mensah, G. A., Alexander, R. W. anderson, J. L., et al. Markers of Inflammation and Cardiovascular Disease: Application to Clinical and Public Health Practice: A Statement for Healthcare Professionals from the Centers for Disease Control and Prevention and the American Heart Association. *Circulation*. 2003; 107: 499–511.

Writing Group for the Women's Health Initiative Investigators. Risks and benefits of estrogen plus progestin in healthy postmenopausal women: Principal results from the Women's Health Initiative randomized controlled trial. *JAMA*. 2002; 288: 321–33.

Women and Heart Disease

Angus, J. The material and social predicaments of home: women's experiences after aortocoronary bypass surgery. *Canadian Journal of Nursing Research*. 2001; 33: 27–42.

Lemolo, F., Martiniuk, A., Steinman, D. A. and Spence, J. D. Sex differences in carotid plaque and stenosis. *Stroke*. 2004; 35: 477–81.

Malacrida, R., Genoni, M. Maggioni, A. P., Spataro, V., et al. A comparison of the early outcome of acute myocardial infarction in women and men. The Third International Study of Infarct Survival Collaborative Group. *New England Journal of Medicine*. 1998; 338: 8–14.

McSweeney, J. C., Cody, M., O'Sullivan, P., Elberson, K., et al. Women's early warning symptoms of acute myocardial infarction. *Circulation*. 2003; 108: 2619–23.

Mosca, L., Appel, L. J., Benjamin, E. J., Berra, K., et al. Evidence-based guidelines for cardiovascular disease prevention in women. *Journal of the American College of Cardiology*. 2004; 43: 900–21.

Natarajan, S., Liao, Y., Cao, G., Lipsitz, S. R. and McGee, D. L. Sex differences in risk for coronary heart disease mortality associated with diabetes and established coronary heart disease. *Archives of Internal Medicine*. 2003; 163: 1735–40.

Schulman, K. A., Berlin, J. A., Harless, W., Kerner, J. F., et al. The effect of race and sex on physicians' recommendations for cardiac catheterization. *New England Journal of Medicine*. 1999; 340: 618–26.

Vaccarino, V., Lin, Z. Q., Kasl, S. V., Mattera, J. A., et al. Sex differences in health status after coronary artery bypass surgery. *Circulation* 2003; 108: 2642–47.

Wenger, N. K., Speroff, L. and Packard, B. Cardiovascular health and disease in women. *New England Journal of Medicine.* 1993; 329: 247–56.

Nutrition and Heart Disease

Appel, L. J., Moore, T. J., Obarzanek, E., Vollmer, W. M., et al. A clinical trial of the effects of dietary patterns on blood pressure. *New England Journal of Medicine.* 1997; 336: 1117–24.

Beveridge, J. M. R., Connell, W. F., Mayer, G. A. and Haust, H. L. Plant sterols, degree of unsaturation and hypocholesterolemic action of certain fats. *Canadian Journal of Biochemistry and Physiology.* 1958; 36: 895–911.

Erkkilä, A. T., Lichtenstein, A. H., Mazaffarian, D. and Herrington, D. M. Fish intake is associated with a reduced progression of coronary-artery atherosclerosis in diabetic women with coronary disease. *American Journal of Clinical Nutrition.* 2004; 80: 626–32.

Hu, F. B., Bronner, L., Willett, W. C., Stampfer, M. J., et al. Fish and omega-3 fatty acid intake and risk of coronary heart disease in women. *Journal of the American Medical Association.* 2002; 287: 1815–21.

Jacobs, D. R., Jr., Meyer, K. A., Kushi, L. H. and Folsom, A. R. Whole-grain intake may reduce the risk of ischemic heart disease death in post-menopausal women: the Iowa Women's Health Study. *American Journal of Clinical Nutrition.* 1998; 68: 248–57.

Joshipura, K. J., Hu, F. B., Manson, J. E., Stampfer, M. J., et al. The effect of fruit and vegetable intake on risk for coronary heart disease. *Annals of Internal Medicine.* 2001; 134: 1106–14.

Kushi, L. H., Sc.D., Folsom, A. R., M.D., Prineas, R. J., M.B., B.S., Mink, P. J., M.P.H., et al. Dietary antioxidant vitamins and death from coronary heart disease in postmenopausal women. *New England Journal of Medicine.* 1996; 334: 1156–62.

Lichtenstein, A. H., Ausman, L. M., Carrasco, W., Jenner, J. L., et al. Short-term consumption of a low-fat diet beneficially affects plasma lipid concentrations only when accompanied by weight loss. Hypercholesterolemia, low-fat diet and plasma lipids. *Arteriosclerosis & Thrombosis.* 1994; 14: 1751–60.

Lichtenstein, A. H., Ausman, L. A., Jalbert, S. M. and Schaefer, E. J. Comparison of different forms of hydrogenated fats on serum lipid levels in moderately hypercholesterolemic female and male subjects. *New England Journal of Medicine* 1999; 340: 1933–40.

Lichtenstein, A. H., Ausman, L. M., Jalbert, S. M., Vilella-Bach, M., et al. Efficacy of a therapeutic lifestyle change/Step 2 Diet in moderately hypercholesterolemic middle-aged and elderly female and male subjects. *Journal of Lipid Research*. 2002; 43: 264–73.

Lichtenstein, A. H., Jalbert, S. M., Adlercreutz, H., Goldin, B. R., et al. Lipoprotein response to diets high in soy or animal protein with and without isoflavones in moderately hypercholesterolemic subjects. *Arteriosclerosis, Thrombosis & Vascular Biology*. 2002; 22:1852–58.

Lichtenstein, A. H. Dietary fat and cardiovascular disease risk: quantity or quality? *Journal of Women's Health*. 2003; 12: 109–14.

Sacks, F. M., Svetkey, L. P., Vollmer, W. M., Appel, L. J., et al. Effects on blood pressure of reduced dietary sodium and the Dietary Approaches to Stop Hypertension (DASH) Diet. DASH-Sodium Collaborative Research Group. *New England Journal of Medicine*. 2001; 344: 3–10.

Schaefer, E. J., Lichtenstein, A. H., Lamon-Fava, S., Contois, J. H., et al. Efficacy of National Cholesterol Education Program Step 2 Diet in normolipidemic and hypercholesterolemic middle-aged and elderly men and women. *Arteriosclerosis & Thrombosis*. 1995; 15: 1079–85.

Schaefer, E. J. Lipoproteins, nutrition and heart disease. *American Journal of Clinical Nutrition*. 2002; 75: 191–212.

Physical Activity and Heart Disease

Gulati, M., Pandey, D. K., Arnsdorf, M. F., Lauderdale, D. S., et al. Exercise capacity and the risk of death in women: the St. James Women Take Heart Project. *Circulation*. 2003; 108: 1554–59.

Mora, S., Redberg, R. F., Cui, Y., Whiteman, M. K., et al. Ability of exercise testing to predict cardiovascular and all-cause death in asymptomatic women: a 20-year follow-up of the lipid research clinics prevalence study. *Journal of the American Medical Association*. 2003; 290: 1600–7.

Blair, S. N., Kampert, J. B., Kohl, H. W., III, Barlow, C. E., et al. Influence of cardiovascular fitness and other precursors on cardiovascular disease and all-cause mortality in men and women. *Journal of the American Medical Association*. 1996; 276: 205–10.

Blair, S. N., Kohl, H. W., 3rd, Paffenbarger, R. S., Jr., Clark, D. G., et al. Physical fitness and all-cause mortality: A prospective study of healthy men and women. *Journal of the American Medical Association.* 1989; 262(17): 2395–401.

Castaneda, C., Layne, J., Munoz-Orians, L., Gordon, P., et al. High-intensity progressive resistance exercise training in Hispanic older adults with type 2 diabetes: a randomized controlled trial. *Diabetes Care.* 2002; 25: 2335–41.

Farrell, S. W., Braun, L., Barlow, C. E., Cheng, Y. J., Blair, S. N. The relation of body mass index, cardiorespiratory fitness and all-cause mortality in women. *Obesity Research.* 2002; 10(6): 417–23.

FitzGerald, S. J., Barlow, C. E., Kampert, J. B., Morrow, J. R., Jr., et al. Muscular fitness and all-cause mortality: prospective observations. *Journal of Physical Activity and Health.* 2004; 1: 7–18.

Hu, F. B., Stampfer, M. J., Colditz, G. A., Ascherio, A., et al. Physical activity and risk of stroke in women. *Journal of the American Medical Association.* 2000; 283(22): 2961–67.

Hu, F. B., Sigal, R. J., Rich-Edwards, J. W., Colditz, G. A., et al. Walking compared with vigorous physical activity and risk of type 2 diabetes in women: a prospective study. *Journal of the American Medical Association.* 1999; 282(15): 1433–39.

Kushi, L. H., Fee, R. M., Folsom, A. R., Mink, P. J., et al. Physical activity and mortality in postmenopausal women. *Journal of the American Medical Association.* 1997; 277(16): 1287–92.

Morris, J. N., Heady, J. A., Raffle, P. A. B., Roberts, C. G. and Parks, J. W. Coronary heart disease and physical activity of work. *The Lancet.* 1953; ii:1053–57.

Paffenbarger, R. S., Jr. Ability of exercise testing to predict cardiovascular and all cause death in asymptomatic women: a 20-year follow-up of the lipid research clinic's prevalence study. *Journal of the American Medical Association.* 2003; 290: 1600–7.

Paffenbarger, R. S., Jr., Wing, A. L. and Hyde, R. T. Physical activity as an index of heart attack risk in college alumni. *American Journal of Epidemiology.* 1978; 108(3): 161–75.

Tanasescu M., Leitzmann M. F., Rimm, E. B., Willett, W. C., et al. Exercise type and intensity in relation to coronary heart disease in men. *Journal of the American Medical Association.* 2002; 288(16): 1994–2000.

Thompson, P. D., Buchner, D, et al. Exercise and physical activity in the pre-
    vention and treatment of atherosclerotic cardiovascular disease: a state-
    ment from the Council on Clinical Cardiology (Subcommittee on
    Exercise, Rehabilitation and Prevention) and the Council on Nutrition,
    Physical Activity and Metabolism (Subcommittee on Physical Activity).
    Circulation. 2003; 107(24): 3109–16.

Complementary Therapies and Heart Disease

Castillo-Richmond, A., Schneider, R. H., Alexander, C. N., Cook, R., et al.
    Effects of stress reduction on carotid atherosclerosis in hypertensive African
    Americans. *Stroke.* 2000; 31(3): 568–73.
King, M. S., Carr, T. and D'Cruz, C. Transcendental Meditation, hyper-
    tension and heart disease. *Australian Family Physicians.* 2002; 31(2):
    164–68.
Liu, E. H., Turner, L. M., Lin, S. X., Klaus, L., et al. Use of alternative medicine
    by patients undergoing cardiac surgery. *Journal of Thoracic and Cardio-
    vascular Surgery.* 2000; 120(2): 335–41.
Spigelski, D. B. and Jones, P. J. H. Efficacy of garlic supplementation in low-
    ering serum cholesterol levels. *Nutrition Reviews.* 2001; 59(7): 236–41.
Zamarra, J. W., Schneider, R. H., Besseghini, I., Robinson, D. K. and Salerno,
    J. W. Usefulness of the Transcendental Meditation programmein the
    treatment of patients with coronary artery disease. *American Journal of
    Cardiology.* 1996; 77(10): 867–70.

Acknowledgements

◆

The names you see on a book cover represent but a small fraction of the people involved in bringing a work to fruition.

We first express our gratitude to Lawrence Bacow, president of Tufts University, for his leadership in bringing nutrition and physical activity to the forefront of the university's mission – and for providing the best example, through his participation in the annual President's Marathon Challenge, of how even the busiest people can find time to take care of themselves through training and eating well.

A number of other present as well as past colleagues at Tufts, many of whom double as close friends, have also buoyed our efforts along the way. Heartfelt appreciation goes to Drs Eileen Kennedy, Irwin Rosenberg, Christina Economos, Jeanne Goldberg, Aviva Must, Raymond Hyatt, Roger Fielding, Ronenn Roubenoff, Carmen Castenada Sceppa, Kristin Baker, Lynne Ausman, Sarah Booth, Arja Erkkila, Nirupa Matthan, Simin Meydan, Ursula Schwab, Susan Roberts and Sonia Vega Lopez. The entire good-hearted staff who work with Miriam at Tufts's John Hancock Center for Physical Activity and Nutrition and with Alice at the Cardiovascular Nutrition Laboratory at the Jean Mayer USDA Human Nutrition Research Center on Aging at Tufts have our sincere gratitude.

A special thanks from Alice to Ernst Schaefer, MD, for the mentoring along with all the encouragement and opportunities he has provided. Also, thanks that can't be adequately expressed in words go to D. Mark Hegsted,

PhD, doctoral thesis adviser to Alice, who has served as a scientific moral role model all these years.

Susan Jalbert must also be mentioned here for single-handedly dealing with all the day-to-day issues of running the Cardiovascular Nutrition Laboratory. There is nothing she wouldn't do to get the job done right. Rebecca Seguin deserves special recognition. She provided invaluable assistance analyzing numerous menus to help us get just right the nutrition programme in this book. We express gratitude as well to Nilda Martin and Lori Ioannone, who ably helped with administrative details. Appreciation also goes to Franci Otting, who served as a model for some of the exercise illustrations.

Many thanks to colleague Daniel Forman, MD, a cardiologist at Harvard Medical School, who graciously agreed to vet this book for us, providing top-notch help with accuracy and details. Any errors that might remain are ours alone.

Of course, without our colleagues at Putnam, none of this could have happened. We salute our editor, Marian Lizzi, for her keen eye and guidance throughout the editing process. And much appreciation goes to all the able individuals in Putnam's publicity department who do their utmost – and always have – to make sure *Strong Women* stays in the news.

Of Wendy Weil, our friend and warmhearted agent, we cannot come up with enough superlatives to thank her for her support through all seven *Strong Women* books. As always, we thank Wendy Wray for her incredible illustrations.

We are indebted to those who fund our research. There are many, but we want to recognize in particular here the National Institutes of Health, the US Department of Agriculture, John Hancock Financial Services, Inc. and the New Balance Foundation.

Individual thanks go from Miriam to Gary Hirshberg at Stonyfield Farms for his help to further the *Strong Women* movement. In addition, Neill Walsdorf Jr. and his colleagues at Mission Pharmacal have greatly enhanced the visibility of *Strong Women* worldwide.

Collaborator Larry Lindner's writing colleagues Gail Zyla, Anne Fletcher, Christine Smith and Mary Thang will never know how important they have been and continue to be. Especially grateful thanks go to Joanna Standley, a young friend with an old soul.

To the people who agreed to be interviewed for this book, thank you for your help in putting voices to the drama of heart disease. Linda, Wendy, Deanne, DeLinda, Kim, Cindy, Helen, Pearl, Judy and Anne have contributed greatly through their candor and patience. So has Nancy Loving, executive director of WomenHeart, who helped put us in touch with some of the women we spoke to.

Larry wishes to thank Shirley Lindner, whose heart is at the heart of everything good; Rochelle and Patricia Lindner, who have been instrumental in bringing joy to our family of men; and the next generation of Lindner women: Kimberly, Heidi, Melanie, Sarah and Amanda. Weren't you all girls just five minutes ago?

As for our spouses, 'thanks' is hardly the word. To Kin Earle, for *always* providing Miriam the support and the freedom that lets her pursue this incredible *Strong Women* journey; to Barry Goldin, for his unwavering confidence in Alice's abilities and for encouraging her to go far beyond what she ever envisioned she could do; and to Constance Lindner. Without Constance, there's no Larry.

Finally, while for obvious reasons this book is dedicated to our daughters, Eliza Earle, Alexandra Earle and Rachel Lichtenstein Goldin, we are equally dedicated to our sons – Mason Earle, David Lichtenstein Goldin and John Lindner. You guys – firstborns, all of you – are the ones who gave us our initial lessons in just how rich and full a heart can grow.

Index

ABOUT THE AUTHORS

Miriam Nelson, PhD, is director of the John Hancock Center for Physical Activity and Nutrition and associate professor of nutrition at the Friedman School of Nutrition Science and Policy, Tufts University. She is also a fellow of the American College of Sports Medicine, an honour reserved for those who have demonstrated leadership and research in the field of exercise.

For the last fifteen years, Dr Nelson has been the principal investigator of studies on exercise and nutrition, work supported by grants from the US government and private foundations. During this time she was named a Brookdale National Fellow, a prestigious award given annually to only five or six young scholars deemed to be future leaders in the field of aging. She was also awarded a Bunting Fellowship at the Mary Ingraham Bunting Institute at Radcliffe College. In 1998, Dr Nelson received the Lifetime Achievement Award from the Massachusetts Governor's Committee on Physical Fitness and Sports.

Dr Nelson is the author of the international best sellers *Strong Women Stay Young*; *Strong Women Stay Slim*; *Strong Women, Strong Bones*; *Strong Women Eat Well*; and *Strong Women* and Men *Beat Arthritis*. She also recently released *The Strong Women's Journal*. These titles, published in fourteen languages, have sold more than a million copies worldwide. *Strong Women, Strong Bones* received the esteemed 'Books for a Better Life Award' for best wellness book of 2000 from the Multiple Sclerosis Society.

In August 2001, Dr Nelson appeared in her own PBS special entitled 'Strong Women Live Well,' which focused on the benefits of exercise and nutrition for women's health. She has been featured on many television and radio shows, including *The Oprah Winfrey Show*, *The Today Show*, *Good Morning America*, ABC Nightly News, CNN, Fresh Air, and the Discovery

Channel. Dr Nelson is a motivational speaker who lectures about women's health around the world. She is also a LLuminari health expert.

She lives in Concord, Massachusetts, with her husband and three children.

Alice H. Lichtenstein, D.Sc., is the Stanley N. Gershoff Professor of Nutrition Science and Policy in the Friedman School at Tufts University, and director of the Cardiovascular Nutrition Laboratory at the Jean Mayer USDA Human Nutrition Research Center on Aging at Tufts. Dr Lichtenstein holds a secondary appointment as professor of family medicine and community health at Tufts University School of Medicine. In June 2005 she will receive an honorary doctoral degree from the Faculty of Medicine, University of Kuopio, Finland.

Dr Lichtenstein has been the principal investigator of numerous National Institutes of Health- and American Heart Association-funded studies addressing the relationship between diet and heart disease risk factors. She has coauthored more than 100 peer-reviewed articles, thirty review articles, and twenty book chapters on nutrition and heart disease and related topics.

Dr Lichtenstein served on the USDA/HHS 2000 Dietary Guidelines Advisory Committee and the Dietary Reference Intake Macronutrient Panel of the National Academy of Sciences, Institute of Medicine, Food and Nutrition Board. She currently serves as chair, Nutrition Committee, American Heart Association. She is also a fellow of the Nutrition, Physical Activity and Metabolism Council and the Arteriosclerosis, Thrombosis and Vascular Biology Council of the American Heart Association. In addition, she is a member of the American Society of Nutritional Sciences and the American Society of Clinical Nutrition.

She has served on the editorial board of the *Journal of Nutrition* and is currently serving on the editorial board of *Atherosclerosis*; as an associate editor for the *Journal of Lipid Research*; and as a member of the editorial advisory boards of the *Journal of Nutrition in Clinical Care* and the *Tufts University Health & Nutrition Letter.* Dr Lichtenstein frequently comments on nutrition-related issues in the popular press, including *The New York Times, Washington Post, Newsweek,* and *Time* magazine. She has also appeared on numerous national television shows, including *The Today Show* and CNN news.

She lives in Newton, Massachusetts, with her husband and two children.

Lawrence Lindner, MA, writes a regular column for the *Boston Globe*. He also penned the 'Eating Right' column for the *Washington Post* for several years and currently freelances for a variety of magazines on health, travel and other subjects. He lives in Hingham, Massachusetts, with his wife and son.

To contact Dr Nelson, please send letters to:
Miriam E. Nelson, PhD
Director, John Hancock Center for Physical Activity and Nutrition
Friedman School of Nutrition Science and Policy
Tufts University
150 Harrison Avenue
Boston, MA 02111
USA

Dr Nelson regrets that, due to the volume of mail she receives, she cannot respond personally to every letter.

Please visit: www.strongwomen.com